Prioritising Child Health

Prioritisation exists throughout healthcare. Difficult and controversial decisions are frequently made at national, local and service level, as well as on an individual basis. However, attention has generally been focused away from the practitioners and service managers who make day-to-day prioritising decisions in order to manage their workloads and deliver front-line services.

Focusing on child health contexts, *Prioritising Child Health* opens up the debate on prioritisation by individuals and explores the issues surrounding their decisions. Key aims of the book are:

- to illustrate prioritisation in practice at different stages in the process of client management
- to review the process of prioritisation from the viewpoint of a range of disciplines
- to develop a new understanding of the process of prioritisation
- to identify principles of good practice for the child health practitioner.

Grounded in the reality of everyday life, *Prioritising Child Health* encourages readers to make their own judgements about how to prioritise. It will appeal to professionals working in child health, including speech and language therapists, occupational therapists and physiotherapists, as well as nurses, doctors and health visitors.

Sue Roulstone is Professor of Speech and Language at the University of the West of England, Bristol and Co-Director of the Speech and Language Therapy Research Unit, Frenchay Hospital, North Bristol Trust.

Prioritising Child Health

Practice and principles

Edited by Sue Roulstone

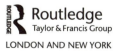

Routledge
Taylor & Francis Group

LONDON AND NEW YORK

First published 2007
by Routledge
2 Park Square, Milton Park, Abingdon, OX14 4RN

Simultaneously published in the USA and Canada
by Routledge
270 Madison Avenue, New York, NY 10016

Routledge is an imprint of the Taylor & Francis Group, an informa business

Typeset in Times New Roman
by Keystroke, 28 High Street, Tettenhall, Wolverhampton
Printed and bound in Great Britain
by MPG Books Ltd, Bodmin, Cornwall

British Library Cataloguing in Publication Data
A catalogue record for this book is available from the British Library

Library of Congress Cataloging in Publication Data
Prioritising child health : practice and principles / edited by Sue Roulstone.
    p. ; cm.
Includes bibliographical references and index.
1. Child health services. 2. Children–Health and hygiene.
I. Roulstone, Sue, 1951– [DNLM: 1. Health Priorities–Great Britain.
2. Professional Role–Great Britain. 3. Child–Great Britain.
4. Decision Making–Great Britain. W 84 FA1 P958 2006]

RJ102.Pa75 2006

362.198'9200941–dc22   2006017392

ISBN10 0–415–37633–5 (hbk)
ISBN10 0–415–37634–3 (pbk)
ISBN10 0–203–96629–5 (ebk)

ISBN13 978–0–415–37633–4 (hbk)
ISBN13 978–0–415–37634–1 (pbk)
ISBN13 978–0–203–96629–7 (ebk)

To 'Katherine', 'James' and 'Thomas', their parents and families

To the many other families that I have met in practice who have to fight for resources for the children

And to the practitioners who are struggling against the odds to provide services.

Contents

Tables and figures

Contributors

Elizabeth J. Croot is Research Fellow, Institute of General Practice and Primary Care, Community Sciences Centre, Northern General Hospital, Sheffield.

Nicola Eaton is Director of Children's Palliative Care Research, Centre for Child and Adolescent Health, University of the West of England, Bristol.

Rosemarie Hayhow is stammering specialist with United Bristol NHS Healthcare Trust, and Senior Research Therapist with the Speech and Language Therapy Research Unit, Bristol.

Tara Kerr-Elliott is Children's Palliative Care Nurse Specialist, Kaleidoscope Team, Kensington and Chelsea Primary Care Trust, London.

Geoff Lindsay is Professor of Special Needs Education and Educational Psychology and Director of the Centre for Educational Development, Appraisal and Research at the University of Warwick.

Michael Loughlin is Reader in Applied Philosophy at Manchester Metropolitan University and Visiting Reader in Philosophy as Applied to Health at Queen Mary's College, London.

Margaret Miers is Professor of Nursing and Social Science, Faculty of Health and Social Care, University of the West of England, Bristol.

Brian Petheram is Reader in Information Systems at the University of the West of England, Bristol and Co-Director of the Speech & Language Therapy Research Unit, Bristol.

Caroline Pickstone is a Research Fellow at the Research Development Support Unit, ScHARR, University of Sheffield and Sheffield Speech and Language Therapy Agency.

Sue Roulstone is Professor of Speech and Language Therapy, Faculty of Health and Social Care, University of the West of England, Bristol, and Co-Director of the Speech and Language Therapy Research Unit, Bristol.

Paul Rowlands is a retired lecturer in economics and management, former business manager in the public sector and consultant to the private sector.

Acknowledgements

I am grateful to all those who have participated in this exploration of prioritisation, particularly Margaret Miers, Brian Petheram and Paul Rowlands, who have supported me with many stimulating discussions during the process of compiling this book, helped me to formulate some of the key arguments of the book, encouraged and enthused when I flagged, and made their own special contributions to the writing. Indeed, I am grateful to all my colleagues who have contributed so thoughtfully and thought-provokingly. My thanks also go to Mr Cliff Warwick and his staff at Trinity Fields School for their help and hospitality. Finally, but most importantly, I'd like to extend my special thanks to the parents who gave their time and stories. Their stories and many like them are the reason I embarked on this project in a desire to understand the problem better and to provide services which make sense to families.

Part I

Introduction

Chapter 1

Why write about prioritisation?

Sue Roulstone

About 20 years ago I took on a post as the 'chief' of a children's speech and language therapy team. The team were under pressure from long waiting lists, and feeling that they were spreading themselves ever thinner and thinner. As a team we tried all kinds of strategies to get this workload under control, with varying levels of success: we tried to increase the staffing levels, by systematic analysis of workloads and workforce planning techniques, prioritisation of different sections of the caseload, working with referral agencies, centralised planning for waiting lists and certain kinds of group work; and when families complained, we directed the complaints (before the new NHS complaints system) through to the upper-level managers of the health authority. Over the years, the nature of the complaints and the source of the pressure points changed, but the problem never really went away.

It led me to the subject of my doctoral thesis, which was to investigate prioritisation of preschool children by speech and language therapists: given that there seemed to be no easy answers in the research literature, I followed the line that the expertise of therapists might somehow be captured and instruct us all. In carrying out my doctoral research, I became aware of how much prioritisation was going on inexplicitly, below the surface of services, never openly discussed with service users and rarely even fed back to higher level management. In researching the literature around prioritisation of speech and language therapy services, I was also aware that little was written on the process for the front-line practitioner. In fact, at the time there were only two references in the field of speech and language therapy: one described a decision process that had been computer generated by case-based analyses (Ward *et al.* 1990) which is in use by one of the authors in this book (Pickstone, chapter 7). The other was a scoring system that allocated points according to the severity of a child's difficulties in the areas of effective communication (Withers 1993). Developed by consensus within the speech and language therapy department, the system provided a severity score. This was, interestingly, not then used to prioritise the most severe children, but to enable therapists to monitor their caseloads and achieve a balanced case load which allowed some throughput of cases, and to demonstrate the caseload weighting and resource needs of different clinics.

During that period (early 1990s) other speech and language therapy research concerning decision making focused on how to define children with communication problems (e.g. Records and Tomblin 1994) and on the process of assessment (e.g. Gerard and Carson 1990) but there was no explicit discussion of prioritisation. In the mid-1990s, the debate about rationing erupted in the medical journals concerning national level rationing. The call came from the medical profession (Lenaghan 1997) for politicians to acknowledge and be accountable for the rationing process. However, nearly a decade later, front-line prioritisation still receives little attention, particularly in healthcare professions other than medicine.

This book aims to fill that gap. It is an expansion of my original research in that it widens the debate beyond speech and language therapy to child health more generally. The aim is to bring some of the pressures that we face into open debate, to explore some of the strategies that are available and in use. This book maintains as its basis a belief that practitioners hold expertise in making these decisions and that exposition and reflection on their decisions can improve the debate about appropriate strategies. Practitioners' and families' experiences therefore provide the setting in Part II of the book.

Prioritisation or rationing?

Prioritisation is a fact of life for us all: whatever we do whenever we act, we make decisions about what we want to do and when, and how many of our resources we wish to commit to any particular activity. In a world of ever-wider choice, we decide how to prioritise our activity, our money and our time. In a healthcare setting, similar prioritising decisions are made and at different levels throughout the system from national government level through and across the system to the individual practitioner (Table 1.1). Of course there is interaction between the various levels. As Lenaghan (1997) notes, 'the challenge is to develop a policy which enables us to define the limits and extent of local flexibility, rather than allowing it to continue to be used as an excuse for all manner of inappropriate variations'. The decisions are complex, with many components, often competing and contradictory. In some fields there is good evidence, general consensus and popular support for prioritising a particular activity in a particular way. Other areas are less certain and potentially controversial.

The word prioritisation is frequently used interchangeably with or instead of a more emotive word: rationing. Rationing is defined by Weale (1995) as 'an implicit or explicit decision to withhold specific measures of treatment or care on the grounds that their economic costs are prohibitive even though the measures in question are thought to yield some . . . benefit'. There have been attempts to distinguish between rationing and priority setting, for example by using rationing to focus on what happens to the individual, and priority setting for the group level (New 1996). The Rationing Agenda Group, set up in 1995 to promote debate on the subject of rationing, chose to use the term 'rationing' deliberately because of its provocative connotations (New 1996). Certainly, in much of the debate about

Table 1.1 Prioritisation decisions, from macro to micro

Where the decision is made	Examples of decisions
National	Is care of the elderly healthcare or social care? Who pays – the NHS or the individual?
	Which treatments will be funded by the NHS? Shall it be hip replacements or cardiac surgery?
Regional	Which services can be provided efficiently and effectively at a local level? (Some will be provided only at a regional level, for example, cochlear implant surgery.)
	To what length of life expectancy will palliative care be funded?
Service	Which schools receive on-site delivery of intervention?
	What proportion of resources should be allocated for continuing professional development?
Team	Should the team work together to provide group interventions or work with children on a one-to-one basis?
	Will the team share out the caseload according to experience and interest or will all the team work with any case?
Individual practitioner	Do I complete my reports or see another child?
	Shall I go to the case conference at another venue or send a report and therefore have time to complete my activity statistics for the week?

national-level services, the word of choice is rationing. In this book we have chosen to use the word prioritisation, in recognition that front-line services and practitioners have no control over macro-level decisions taken about the overall level of resources allocated to their sector and that the decisions they make are about the control of resources for individuals; this can of course still mean the exclusion of certain individuals and groups from services. We recognise that this distinction is tenuous (see Chapter 9, note 6); however, in part, we have opted to use the term because it seems to be the term of frequent use in practice contexts.

As indicated, much of what has been written about rationing focuses on national-level decisions, the macro level, although there are occasional forays into what happens at the meso and micro levels. The writings can be summed up under the gloss of 'trying to work out how to prioritise in a fair and equitable manner'. Researchers and writers comment on the variability of healthcare and the lack of consensus not only about which care groups should be prioritised but also about the criteria used to prioritise. All acknowledge the complexity of the problem and the unlikelihood of a simple solution. Typically, there is a search not for agreement about the criteria for rationing but for a set of 'constraining . . . principles' (Weale 1995) which can be brought to bear on the decision-making process. Weale, for example, discusses the rationale and implications of considering effectiveness, efficiency, fairness and democratic responsiveness.

A changing context for decision making

During the period of my research there have been many changes that influence how decisions are being made within child health and the wider healthcare system. As part of the exploration of the rationale for this book, it is useful to consider some of these, in particular: the changing nature of professional power and authority, increased accountability and user involvement in decision making.

The changing nature of professional power and authority

Traditional views accepted that professionals had the best interests of their patients at heart and could not only be trusted and relied upon to make the right decisions for their patients, but were above the challenge of their patients. My parents' generation considered it unthinkable and downright discourteous to question the doctor, even if they may have been dissatisfied and 'non-compliant' with the services. Over the last generation, professional power and status have been challenged and eroded. The information revolution is making a contribution to this changing picture. The public now has access to a full range of information and support groups through the internet, enabling them to challenge the once-exclusive knowledge of the healthcare practitioner. Government has also contributed to this shift in its policy work, promoting the notion of patient choice (DoH 2003b), the expert patient (DoH 2000), and 'full engagement' of patients in their own healthcare (Wanless 2004). Paley (2006) argues that the evidence-based practice movement also has the potential to change the power of experts: since information is power, it will be those who are familiar with and able to interpret the evidence base who will be able to exert power over decisions in the future. These people are not necessarily those whose expertise is based in clinical experience and positions of power in the system.

Increased accountability

The increasing challenge from the public to public sector workers generally and to the healthcare sector in particular, requires that practitioners and their managers are able to justify and rationalise their decisions and be accountable for their actions. This trend has been accentuated over the last decade as a result of a number of high-profile cases where the medical profession has failed to live up to the expectation of acting in the best interests of their patients (Bristol Royal Infirmary Inquiry 2000, Royal Liverpool Children's Hospital Inquiry 2001; Shipman Inquiry 2002). These changes have not only affected the medical profession but have had an impact across the healthcare system. Alongside the escalating costs of healthcare, the need to control healthcare practitioners has generated the introduction of a range of quality management techniques, including standard setting, clinical governance and service monitoring that have been implemented across wide sectors of healthcare, including research.

User involvement

A related agenda is that of increasing the contribution of the public and service user in healthcare decision making. Within my own profession and others involved in child health, the involvement of parents in the assessment and provision of interventions for their child has always predominated – at least since I qualified in the early 1970s. However, our understanding and approach has changed over that time, informed by a general development of policy and research on the subject, and the notion of involvement has evolved into one of partnership. Our understanding of how to involve children is still very new and relatively untried although it, too, is now embedded in the Government's policy agenda (DoH 2003a).

The involvement of the public or patients in decision making can take place at many levels in the planning and delivery of services (Tritter et al. 2003) but is clearly not a straightforward or easy process. New (1996), for example, points out the varying values held by different members of society and asks how we should weight decisions to reflect the views of a particular group. The parents in a study of speech and language therapy services varied in their attitudes towards the process of early identification (Glogowska and Campbell 2004). Patients are already engaged in the process of prioritisation with health authorities (Gold 2005) and accept the need for prioritisation to occur, but perceive a need for improved explanation and information about the process and system and the alternatives that might be available (Cross et al. 2006). Finally, it is likely that patients (and in the case of child health, probably parents) will vary as to the level at which they wish to be involved in decision making. Dowie (2002) suggests that a patient's preferred relationship with a doctor will vary around three functions: the level of decision-making responsibility, the amount of information provided and value clarification required.

Prioritisation in action

Part II of this book presents stories and examples from families and from practitioners about their everyday experiences in child health. The stories are illustrative, intended to draw you into the topic area and to ground subsequent discussions in real life. We start with stories from the mothers of three children with various disabilities. These are transcripts of interviews that I conducted. Each mother has read and approved the transcript and chosen a pseudonym for their child. Each starts with a description of their child and I am struck by the normality of these loving descriptions. The stories tell of the highs and lows, the joys and struggles of their life supporting their child. Two of the children have quite rare disabilities and all the children are now teenagers. Child health practices have changed since these parents first struggled to find a diagnosis for their children. Perhaps some of the paternalistic practices they describe will have changed since these children were small. Yet their stories would still be recognised in part by parents of younger children facing those challenges. I could, for example, have asked a parent I know whose son has autism to tell his story of fighting for speech and language therapy in school. Or I could have asked the parent who would like the opinion of an occupational therapist for her clumsy child to tell of their time on the waiting lists. And the ongoing difficulties of maintaining continuity of services at points of transition are well known. So, the stories told here are not meant to be exhaustive or even representative, merely illustrative and real.

Similarly, the examples from practitioners do not cover all disciplines within child health. We hear from a children's palliative care nurse, a physiotherapist and, from my own profession, speech and language therapists. They describe a situation in their practice in which prioritisation is occurring in some way. Their descriptions provide an account of the situation as they see it, what the prioritisation action has been and an evaluation of that action. The examples cover day-to-day decisions about managing a workload, team responses to changes in staffing resources, a service-wide approach to ensuring equity of access and a specialist practitioner sharing her expertise of a disorder. While practitioners reading these examples may not find their own discipline represented, they should find examples that have resonance with some aspect of their own practice.

Perspectives from theory

Part of my personal quest is to understand what is happening in healthcare, how we make decisions and how the process of service provision might be improved. I like to ask people who have different perspectives and different theoretical glasses through which to gaze for their views. The differences they bring can add new insights. The parents' perspective at the beginning of the book gives us the starting points and the practitioners put their perspective. In Part III, four authors from differing theoretical perspectives write about prioritisation from the perspective of their discipline. The first of these 'theory' chapters is written, rather reluctantly, by a philosopher, Michael Loughlin. I will leave him to explain his reluctance. Loughlin challenges some of our basic assumptions – even that the use of theory in this way can be helpful. He questions the assumption that the context in which we work is a given that we cannot challenge and the usefulness of the theorists to practitioners faced with inadequate resources. The philosophical frame stimulates us to question each word for what it betrays of the writer's underlying ideology. Starting off the 'theory' chapters in this way gives us a health warning about how to read the rest of the book.

Our second contributor, Margaret Miers, moves our thinking away from the direct focus on prioritisation and rationing to the underlying process of decision making and professional judgement. Miers provides us with an overview of the process of professional judgement and the factors which influence us and outlines some of the decision analytical tools that are available to support the decision-making process.

When we hear the word economics, most of us think of money and the Chancellor directing the economy in Whitehall. But the study of economics is not just about money but the examination of behaviour in terms of how individuals or groups handle resources. In Chapter 11, Paul Rowlands strips out the complexity of the subject of economics and considers basic economic concepts that are appropriate to and therefore can help us to think about prioritisation through yet another set of spectacles.

Finally in Chapter 12, Geoff Lindsay provides a perspective from education. The children we work with in health spend a large proportion of their time in an education context. Decisions made about how healthcare services are offered impact upon their education and their time in school. Lindsay looks at some of the conflicts that can arise between health and education and describes a range of factors that an educationist finds important in prioritising children for services.

Final reflections

The book is rather like a research process: it begins with some background reflections, presents data collected from a number of sources and then considers the possible meaning of that data before drawing conclusions. Chapter 13 is a discussion chapter in which Brian Petheram and I draw together the main themes from the book and discuss the questions they seem to raise. The title of the book includes the phrase 'Practice and Principles' so you might expect that by Chapter 13 some definitive principles would be appearing. In my naivety and optimism, I had hoped that that might indeed be possible. However, we have entitled the chapter 'some answers questioned' in recognition of the fact that we have ended with at least as many questions as we started – quite typical of the research process, in fact! However the final reflections of Chapter 14 conclude that the book fulfils its aims: to open the debate and provide a range of ways of thinking about prioritisation.

References

Bristol Royal Infirmary Inquiry (2000) *The inquiry into the management of care of children receiving complex heart surgery at the Bristol Royal Infirmary*. Interim report: London: HMSO.

Cross, E., Goodacre, S. and O'Cathain, A. J. (2006) 'Rationing in the emergency department: the good, the bad, and the unacceptable', *Emergency Medical Journal*, **22**: 171–6.

Department of Health (2000) *The Expert Patient: A New Approach to Chronic Disease Management for the 21st Century*. London: Department of Health.

Department of Health (2003a) *Every Child Matters*. London: Department of Health.

Department of Health (2003b) *Building on the best: choice, responsiveness and equity in the NHS*. London: Department of Health.

Dowie, J. (2002) 'The role of patients' meta-preferences in the design and evaluation of decision support systems', *Health Expectations* **5(2)**: 156–71

Gerard, K.A. and Carson, E.R. (1990) 'The decision making process in child language assessment', *British Journal of Disorders of Communication*, **25(1)**: 61–75.

Glogowska, M. and Cambell, R. (2004) 'Parental views of surveillance for early speech and language difficulties', *Children and Society*. **18**: 266–77.

Gold, M.R. (2005) 'Tea, biscuits and healthcare prioritizing', *Health Affairs*, **24 (1)**: 234–9.

Lenaghan, J. (1997) 'The rationing debate: central government should have a greater role in rationing decisions – the case for', *British Medical Journal* **314**: 967.

New, B. (1996) 'The rationing agenda in the NHS', *British Medical Journal*, **312**: 1593–601.

Paley, J. (2006) Evidence and expertise. Paper presented at a philosophy seminar, University of the West of England, Bristol.

Records, N.L. and Tomblin, J.B. (1994) 'Clinical decision making: describing the rules of practising speech-language pathologists', *Journal of Speech and Hearing Disorders*, **37**: 144–56.

Royal Liverpool Children's Hospital Inquiry (2001) *Summary and recommendations*. London: Crown Copyright.

Shipman Inquiry (2002) *Death Disguised*. First report. London. (Chair Dame Janet Smith DBE).

Tritter, J., Daykin, N., Evans, S. and Sanidas, M. (2003) *Improving cancer services through patient involvement*. Oxford: Radcliffe Medical Press.

Wanless Report (2004) *Securing good health for the whole population*. London: HMSO.

Ward, S., Birkett, D. and Kellet, B. (1990) 'An expert way of prioritizing clients', *Speech Therapy in Practice* **5(11)**: 12.

Weale, A. (1995) 'The ethics of rationing', *British Medical Bulletin*, **51(4)**: 831–41.

Withers, P. (1993) 'Making children a priority', *College of Speech and Language Therapists Bulletin*, **498** (January): 12–13.

Part II

Prioritisation in action

Chapter 2

Katherine

Katherine is sixteen now. She's tall, very pretty. She's quiet, especially with people she's not familiar with, but at home, she rules the roost. She's very stubborn. She doesn't like being asked or requested to do anything. She's very adamant that she's not going to do it if she doesn't want to do it. She's got a lot of good qualities. She's very happy, she's got a lovely smile and, as I said, she's very pretty. I love her to bits but she really is a madam and she knows what buttons to press with me. Katherine is a healthy girl. She's an excellent swimmer. She's won lots of medals for swimming. She's good on the computer as well. Katherine is her own person I think. Katherine's got two older brothers, 21 and 19, so she's the only granddaughter. She is a bit spoilt by us and the rest of the family because she's the only girl.

She's got very complex difficulties and she's got a condition called tubero-sclerosis (TS) with associated epilepsy and learning disabilities. What the condition means is that she's got tuber-like growths within her brain. And these growths, depending on where they're located in the brain, they cause certain problems, like Katherine's epilepsy, learning disability, her speech and language is affected and, like I say, she has behavioural problems as well. Thankfully, her motor skills are fine. These tubers, they can appear anywhere in the body, even behind the eyes, the kidneys and the heart. They can affect the skin as well. Katherine has a facial rash which starts on her nose and goes right out to her cheekbones . . . it's called a butterfly rash, and can spread down around her mouth and chin as well and also has a patch on her forehead. For the facial rash she's having laser treatment, which is quite successful and it's reduced it quite a lot.

She's monitored on a six-monthly basis by the ophthalmology department . . . because these tubers that can grow behind the eyes are very slow growing and she has been monitored for that for several years but they were so pleased with her . . . that they discharged her. They said if they were going to appear, they would have appeared by now, by age 14. So she is seen locally by the optician and the agreement is that if the optician is worried in any way, that she will be referred back to them.

She has got these tumours on her kidneys but they are harmless at the moment. She has a scan on them every two years to see if they have grown. She's monitored by the cardiology department . . . as well. She has got something suspicious on her heart. It's not interfering with the functioning of her heart but it's there. They don't want to see her until she's eighteen now to see how it's developed and all her services are co-ordinated by a paediatrician. . . . I must say she's really good and has been very good to us . . . we've got an open door policy with her. She monitors Katherine's seizures and prescribes her medication.

How did the diagnosis come about?

Well, it was very traumatic. After having two boys I knew that there was something not right with Katherine. Couldn't pinpoint quite what but I knew there was something different. She used to scream a lot, used to draw her legs up as if in pain and her arms used to thrash out. She used to be quite vacant as well. I was back and forward to the GP for months, trying to tell them that there was something wrong and they kept telling me that I was a paranoid mother, that it was only colic and she will grow out of it. And this was going on for months and months . . . still kept going back until I became so desperate that I went to see another doctor within the practice. She said she didn't think there was anything to worry about but she would make a referral to a consultant anyway.

So a referral was made and took some time to be processed and it was a week before her first birthday that we had an appointment with this consultant . . . and by history she knew there was something not quite right as well and said she would like to do some more tests. So we went down and she had an EEG to monitor the brain activity and that came back abnormal and showing signs of epilepsy so they said that they would like to do a CAT scan. So we agreed to that and she had to be sedated for that. And then we had the results that evening that it was TS.

It was devastating.

The consultant came over to see us and said that had he realised the severity of the child's condition then he would have seen her immediately. I was very cross with the GP and have changed to another practice. I mean, what Katherine has got, she's got, and nothing can be done about it but time was of the essence really and I'll never forgive them for that. My opinion is that if you don't know, ask someone who does. It was a week before her first birthday that we were told that she might never walk, never talk, never do anything but she has proved them wrong.

I've been fighting for speech and language therapy for about twelve, thirteen years. She's got a statement which clearly that says that she requires speech and language input cos her needs are quite complex, but there was just no therapists about. In the end we wrote a letter to a local MP and had a meeting with him and as a result of that speech therapy was provided at the school. Then, she wasn't at that school long then, she had to move on . . . to another school and they didn't have speech and language therapy provision either. And of course, it was out of county as well . . . comes under a different borough, but again there was no input there so we had to keep pushing for it. There's no transition at all from one school to another, it's a nightmare. We did have a therapist but they came and went as they do. They were assessing Katherine, providing a programme and then the classroom staff were implementing the programmes. And then, she was transferred to this school then and the same thing happened here, I only phoned [the headteacher] up on Monday to see what was happening. She did eventually have an assessment back in January but I still haven't had a report for that. Still waiting for a programme even though the classroom staff are marvellous, they actually implement the programme which works well but it doesn't seem to be monitored by the therapist. She doesn't communicate with me, although saying that she did write a note in the book . . . As long as I know what's happening I don't mind but it's the not knowing.

The programmes are devised around Katherine's needs. As I say, they are complex and when a programme is being implemented I feel it needs to be monitored to see that the programme is doing the job that it is supposed to be doing. If it's not working for Katherine then it will need to be adjusted. There is no feedback either, nor re-assessments to see if any progress has been made. It's not consistent. It's a very poor service.

What would make things better?

In an ideal world, I would like to meet the person and I would like the person to meet Katherine and get to know her. Play games and do things that Katherine enjoys doing before she actually did the assessment so Katherine would have a bond with her. When the assessment took place then perhaps I wouldn't be present but I would be about so that I could contribute anything. I would like to have a report of the findings of the assessment and give an input. And have an opportunity to discuss it. And then when the programme goes into place to be able to see the programme, see what's happening, what's working and have a say really. Then when further assessment is done see what progress has been made. There was a speech and language therapy assistant here a few years ago and she was very good, and she was implementing the programme and she used to do fun things with Katherine . . . it was all age appropriate . . . but then she moved on and the classroom support staff have sort of taken over now. They are very good as well mind, but, they don't seem to have any continuity at all. I just feel as if I was pushed from pillar to post.

What about other health services?

Katherine has very complex behavioural problems and we are waiting to see a psychiatrist. We had a psychiatric nurse come out to our house who did an assessment. What she said she would do is take it back to the doctor . . . and they would have like a case conference and it would be decided how it would be best how to handle Katherine's problem . . . whether it would just be nurse input or support staff but I had a letter back just after Christmas to say that [the doctor] will actually see her at her clinic. What the waiting list is or how long that will take I don't know.

[The psychiatric nurse] did explain [about the case conference]. She was very nice. She gave me a card with her contact number on if I ever needed her. Unless she's got a magic wand there's no more we can do. We have been plodding along like this for years and you just get used to it. I don't like it because her behaviour is so awful at home but what can I do about it? . . . I'm willing to try anything. She's always had behavioural problems in the past. I thought it was just part and parcel of her condition.

I think the main thing for me is communication. There just doesn't seem to be any communication between professionals and parents but I think as long as us parents know what's going on, I can accept that, it's the not knowing. Chasing people up all the time. We have enough to do. You don't need to be chasing like we are . . . it's very wearing like I said because you have to be on your toes all the time I feel . . . I feel that Katherine is my priority. If I don't fight for her rights then there's no-one else who will do it for me. I just want her to have the best. So that she can develop to the best of her potential. If that means fighting for a service that she's rightfully entitled to then that's the way it's going to be . . . I am willing to do that for her.

On a more positive note, the consultant that Katherine sees, we get a very good service from her. There was an incident back in February, Katherine had a very nasty seizure in the morning and she fell out of a chair and had a head injury. We needed an ambulance and she was taken to hospital. She was fine when she got there but they suggested that we saw her own consultant because she's on medication so we came home and I phoned [the consultant's] secretary in the afternoon, she said, leave it with me, and later that afternoon she phoned me back, and said we could see [the consultant] in the morning and that's a brilliant service. And she co-ordinates Katherine's health services, like she does the kidney scans, the heart scans, and when she is seen by the various health professionals they all write back to her, so she co-ordinates it all.

She's the medic that I respect and trust. She's just a friendly nice professional. She knows her stuff and Katherine's been seeing her for many years and I've got faith in her. I think [the trust has] developed over the years, the service she's provided for Katherine. The way that she speaks to me, she gives me eye contact.

I've met some health professionals and all they're interested in is writing on a bit of paper, they don't give you eye contact. And your opinions don't matter. [The consultant] asks my opinion . . . what's happening with Katherine, she looks at me and takes time to listen. [She] is someone to turn to because you know when you're out on a limb like that, with this really complex condition when such a lot of things can go wrong, it's just nice to have someone you know you can turn to. And we've got an open door policy so you can just ring up and go.

As I said, Katherine is seen locally now by an optician and she's very good and she's aware of the condition. She's good, it's not a problem. Because of Katherine's lack of ability to wait, patience to wait, in the waiting room she will always see Katherine first, first appointment in the afternoon after school. So that's good. They have obviously taken on board her difficulties. Regarding dentists, that was a bit of an issue, she wouldn't wait in the waiting room in an ordinary dentist, it seemed like a very long wait, by the time she got in there then she just lost it, so I had a word with the dentist, the local dentist, and she said she would make a referral to the school which is much better, she goes along with the rest of the children, and the dentist, she's very good at communicating and she will write me a letter if there's anything to say, she'll give me a ring, so communication there is very good.

Chapter 3

James

James is the youngest of three boys. Very bubbly. He seems very confident but he can be quite shy and quite nervous with people he's [meeting] for the first time. Very talkative, he's always got something to say. When he's adorable, he is adorable, but when the mood takes him he can be really nasty. His language at times is atrocious. I sometimes wonder where he picks up words like that. He gets on well with both of his brothers. His older brother more so – they have quite a strong relationship. He is quite sporty, he is quite good at running, he's won medals for 100m and 200m. He enjoys swimming. If James is out, he is enjoying himself. He enjoys going out to places to eat, that's one of his favourite pastimes. He seems to know all the best restaurants and cafés so his class teacher has informed us. He gets on well with all of the children in his class and has a good relationship with the teachers. He's fifteen.

He was diagnosed with a condition called FG syndrome when he was twelve, which really means there's problems with learning, severe learning difficulties. There's issues with physical development. He's got epilepsy which they say is not always part of the condition. He was born with the centre part of his brain missing, so in James's words he's got two brains. That doesn't help his co-ordination very well.

I knew from the day he was born there was something not right. He had similar facial deformities that his older cousin had. My husband couldn't see it at all, but I could see that within his face he had huge dimples in his temples. When he was about 4 months old my neighbour asked me what was wrong with his ear. He's got a low-set ear on his left side and she said 'Is it curled over?' and I said 'No, that's just him.' Constantly from the day he came out of hospital he projectile vomited. We went to see the GP on numerous occasions. We could see he wasn't developing as well as a baby of his age should be. I was told I was paranoid, I was told that I had postnatal depression and that I was imagining that there was things wrong with the child and there wasn't. And one evening he projectile vomited and my husband said 'Take that baby back to the doctor tomorrow' and I said 'No you take him'. . . . I insisted my husband took him because I felt that the GP didn't believe what I was saying. My husband took time off work. That afternoon we had a phone call from the hospital to say that we had got an appointment that week and we took him to the hospital and the doctor that we seen said 'All babies are sick, there is nothing wrong with him. We will see how he is in six months.' He continued to projectile vomit and we took him back again and we got another appointment that was a week later. We took him to the hospital and they said to us 'Right we'll show you where his bed is', and we said 'He is not staying in we've just come up for the visit', and they said 'No we are keeping him in'. I stayed in with James and [my husband] went home, and the nurse turned around to me and said 'Your husband's very aggressive, isn't he' and I said 'No he's very concerned and very upset because of the way we've been treated'.

A professor came to see James that week and he came into the room and picked up one leg and dropped it and said 'This baby's got no tone' and I asked him what that means, and he said 'I'm very concerned'. Still we didn't have a diagnosis because nobody knew what was happening. We spent the next five, six months going back and forth to the hospital, being weighed, measured, his head circumference was growing alarmingly, as the rest of his body wasn't. And in the November we went to see this professor again, basically, he said 'We have done all the tests, the brain scan, we've done the CAT scan'. He said 'take your baby home and love him as much as you can'. Still no explanation why but he would never move from that position. My husband turned round and said, 'I want a second opinion.' We seen another consultant and from the November to the January we had a series of hearing tests, physiotherapy sessions . . . the consultant arranged them.

[By this time] James was sixteen months old. He could not sit up, couldn't do anything basically. In our view, [the new consultant] was our lifesaver because he acknowledged there was something wrong with James but there could be something done. We were there for two and a half years, he actually kitted out James with grommets and just after he had the grommets we suddenly realised he had a voice, and this deep voice came out. His father and I just sat there and cried because we'd heard his voice, he was about two and all of a sudden we heard his voice.

We were seen by genetics because of my nephew and they mentioned FG syndrome but they sent all the files to the person who specialised in FG syndrome. This was when he was two . . . the report comes back saying no they haven't got FG syndrome, full stop.

We moved [to another area]. The very first visit [to the hospital] we seen a consultant, she started off, 'We can't do this for him, we can't do that for him'. I just got up and walked out in tears. When I composed myself I came back in and my husband said 'We don't want to hear this, what we want to hear is what you can do for us'. He said we've spent over 12 months being told things can't be done. From then on she endeavoured to do her best for us.

He walked just after he was three. He had input from physiotherapy usually in six week blocks then he'd have a break. He developed very slowly.

After another move the family are registered with another consultant paediatrician

We were referred then to a community paediatrician. We were happy to begin with but then we got very disillusioned with the care James was receiving so we asked for a new referral and we actually see [another community paediatrician] now and she was very, very helpful.

Why were you disillusioned with the services?

We had to fight for everything. If we were concerned about something with James we were either fobbed off or it was 'Well, we'll see how he goes before we refer him somewhere else.' We were more concerned about his legs because he had a lot of pain in his legs and there were concerns about his spine curving and without really examining him she dismissed it so we felt very disillusioned with that.

[Then] we went to see [the next paediatrician] and we've been there now two, two and a half years and her view was completely different. 'If you're at all worried just phone me, if there is anything we can do we will check it out.' Since then, she's examined his back, and she says that there is a slight curve in it and she's arranged for physiotherapy for his legs and to check his back. It's just they are more positive. More so as a mother I see more things than even his father sees and I felt our views were being taken on board.

Talking about physiotherapy

They identified he had a need and there were classes, physiotherapy classes with a group of children and we done exercises with them in a fun way that was appropriate to all the children but if the one child needed something a bit more it would be adapted to that one child. Very, very friendly atmosphere. In the very early days, I would say three of the five week days he was at some sort of therapy and there were no issues at all. Then, in [particular area], it wasn't that good. When we moved [to current house] the physiotherapy was good. Within six months of moving here, he had specialised equipment, seating equipment, cutlery, which I never even thought of in [previous home] and it was certainly never on offer, we just muddled through. Down here, they were more forthcoming with help.

We saw a consultant down here and she asked us if we could refer him to another consultant because she was very concerned with his eyesight, with a problem with his eye. When I pushed to find out what it was, she said 'Oh, nothing to worry about' but she was very concerned but for a parent it was 'There's nothing to worry about' which worries me more then. When we seen the consultant I did ask him and he said his viewing wasn't quite right and they were monitoring him to see if it was getting any worse and then they discharged him after about two years with a view that if we were ever worried, if he showed any signs of abnormal behaviour with his eyes you could always take him back.

What would have made things better?

I think people being more open. As I've said, I'm a big believer that parents know best. I think if professionals were more open and explained, not in their terminology but in terminology that I would understand, I would feel much happier. I wouldn't worry so much. The geneticist we see is extremely helpful. I actually found FG syndrome on the internet, I took all the information to the geneticist and said to her 'What do you think?' and I said it was mentioned when he was two and I can see at least ten things that James has got. She said 'What I'll do is send all of James's notes and all my nephew's notes to America to the doctor who first diagnosed it.' Within six months we had a diagnosis back and I felt that she was really listening to our views.

At the moment we are on an ongoing saga. He's had toothaches since February and we have been waiting to have his teeth taken out. If he hadn't had any problems at all he'd have gone down the end of February, been booked into the clinic and had his teeth out. Because he's got complex medical needs, he can't just have a tooth out. He has to go to hospital and have a general anaesthetic. So we were told he was going to go on the waiting list and it was going to be a month. Then he started having toothache and we were sent to another department to see an anaesthetist. She wasn't happy to do it there and then. At the moment it's just so frustrating because he is in so much pain with toothache and yet my other son, we weren't even living down here at the time, he had an abscess and he had his tooth taken out that day because there are no medical problems wrong with him.

I think there should be an emergency list for children that have medical problems so that they can go straight in and have the treatment they need instead of drawing it out. They don't understand what's going on, he gets very frustrated. Every time I take him to the dentist it's 'Do I have to have a needle?' and I can't say yes or no because I don't know.

Chapter 4

Thomas

His name is Thomas. He is seventeen. He is the middle of the three boys. From birth, the heaviest of all three. Emergency caesarean, as the other two were. No health issues initially . . . bouncing baby boy, great appetite, there was nothing to say there was anything wrong. Then when he was seven months old I was very concerned because he wasn't making any sounds. I actually asked the health visitor if she could do the hearing test, but it was before he was seven months old. And she said 'Well do you want a full scale conversation with him?' I said 'No but I'm getting to the stage I'm thinking of putting a bell round his neck to know where he is,' because he would crawl everywhere and not make a sound. She referred him to an audiologist and he failed his hearing test.

Then when he was six months old he suddenly stopped growing lengthways. Piled on the weight but he didn't grow lengthwise. The health visitor came back 'We're very concerned he hasn't grown', so I was already pregnant with [third child] at the time so you can imagine my hormones. Thinking well I've got this perfect bouncing baby boy and suddenly been bombarded with these problems. We were referred to a paediatrician who did bone X-rays on his wrists and ankles with the advice to 'wait until the new baby's born, if he hasn't grown by then we'll talk about growth hormones'. He grew half an inch in that six months. My theory was I'm not very tall, his dad's just touching six foot so that's not excessively tall so I wasn't that worried.

Still with some babbling but not much. It didn't help that my first born seemed to come out talking and he seemed to talk from such an early age and he was very precise with what he was saying, you could understand things at a very early age. When [James] was two he was referred to a speech therapist and we done a six-week session and she said 'Well I don't think there's anything that wrong with him.' Still failed his hearing tests, so that was really ongoing.

He was, we thought, mischievous from the day he turned one. It was like switching on and he was into everything. We weren't that concerned about it. Whereas his older brother would sit down and colour and draw things out – never interested him at all, . . . that was OK.

He was about just under 4 when we moved . . . Still not very good at speech and what speech he had, I could barely understand him and other people couldn't understand him at all. Very much a loner, he wanted to play on his own and sit for hours with cars. We came down here on holiday and my sister's neighbour asked if he was autistic. And I just thought that that was so silly.

When he went off to school when he was rising five and I asked for speech therapy. A friend of his was having speech therapy and they said they would tag him on with him and they had lessons together. When the boy's therapy finished so Thomas's finished regardless of whether he needed it or not, it finished. Still failing his hearing test, no explanation for it.

In school, the teachers all said that he was OK. There is social issues . . . if he wanted a red pencil he would take the red pencil regardless if another child was colouring, he just took it. Still, we were not aware of any concerns. At parenting things [teachers said] 'He's doing OK, nothing to worry about.' That's all we kept having.

Then we moved here, and for the first two years he was fine, nothing to worry about and the breakthrough was a special needs teacher . . . actually started teaching Thomas's class. She rang me up one day and said 'Could you come into school and have a word?' Went into school, she says 'Do you realise that Thomas has got . . . learning difficulties?' and I said 'Well what do you mean?' So she showed me his work and what I could read of it, if he was unsure of anything he would put his name instead of the word. And so we'd be reading a story what he had wrote and it would be 'Thomas' right the way through. 'Have you any explanation' and she says 'Well . . . we call it specific learning difficulties'. I said 'I don't care what you call it'. Because when both boys started school, every school they went to we made them aware that their father has dyslexia and if they show any signs at all, we would like it picking up as soon as possible, not waiting and seeing. Apparently X Education Authority does not acknowledge dyslexia as a specific learning difficulty so it was never picked up there. This teacher then said she wanted him assessed, and I said, 'Oh please, do whatever you have to do'. We'd had behavioural issues with him, very frustrated, very violent at times, it would take a lot but when he exploded, he exploded. Well, she said 'Right, we'll get this assessment done' and it came back and he had a reading age of six years, a spelling age of six years and one month and a comprehension age of thirteen years and one month, this was when he was nine years and two months.

In the meantime his behaviour was extreme and he was doing odd behaviour as we call it. And we were referred to [a paediatrician] and her initial reaction, this was when he was twelve, 'He is a teenager, what do you expect?' What he had done, we had some blinds in his bedroom, vertical blinds, when I looked the string had been cut on the side and I said to him 'What's happened?' and he sat there and never took his eyes off what he was doing and he would swear and that was plain and simple, he needed string, the string was there, simple, to us it was, 'well didn't you think that Mum and Dad would go mad?' 'But I needed string' and it was rational to him. I said to my husband 'This isn't right, this is odd', and there were other incidences. He was different from his older brother. He would smash things up right from an early age he would take things apart just to see how they work.

We were referred to a psychiatrist which really didn't help. . . . Meanwhile, his behaviour was getting worse and worse. He was fighting constantly with his brothers and out of sheer frustration, he wanted to kill himself and as you can imagine it was really upsetting. He would get himself in such a state, he was useless, 'With this dyslexia I can't do anything,' 'I'm no use to anyone'.

I asked 'Has he got ADHD' and we filled out all the forms and he was assessed, and told 'No', I was trying to think of an explanation for his behaviour and it kept being thrown back in my face, 'no, no, no'. And then, we were seeing [the paediatrician] and I felt the visits weren't as worthwhile as they could have been because I felt I was ending up in tears because I was so frustrated, trying to get help, and the doctor basically told me that I was the problem and that I have a totally different relationship with Thomas than I do with the two children and that was why Thomas's behaviour was as bad as it was, that I didn't give him enough praise or talked to him and I felt at my lowest low.

We saw the occupational therapist in October . . . and she said 'From what I've seen today, I don't think he's got anything wrong with him, but I need to speak to someone senior and we need to look at his past records'. Within a week she had rung me back, she said 'I don't know how to explain this to you, he's got developmental co-ordination disorder' and I said 'What's that?', she said 'Well, it used to be called dyspraxia'. How he slipped through the net when he was twelve I don't know and I felt very, very let down. He's come this far without really any real support and it wasn't because we were uncaring parents. We actually took him back to see [the doctor] and she said 'Oh yes, it's developmental co-ordination disorder, oh yes I can understand that' and I felt well if she could understand that why couldn't you have seen it when we first brought him? I feel everything we have needed for Thomas hasn't been there and what we have got for him we have had to push for which I found very frustrating.

I sometimes think it's because I'm an anxious mum anyway, whether I don't get my view across as well as I'd like to. A lot of times if there's something important that I need to get across I'd say to my husband, 'Take time off work and come with me, because they listen to you better'. It's not so much that they listen to him better, he's able to put across what we want to say better.

With Thomas if you'd seen him walking down the street you wouldn't think there was anything at all wrong. He does most things that a seventeen-year-old boy would do, and because he coped in mainstream school, although he's had the support of a support worker with his English work I don't think people really take it seriously. People think there can't be much wrong with him if he's doing A levels. What they don't see is that to enable him to get the grades in GCSE to do sixth form he had to have some of his writing exams done for him and someone to read them. So literally sat there and told them the answers, but a lot of people don't see that. And I think with dyslexia and dyspraxia it's the hidden disabilities, as I call them. In health issues and social services issues, he doesn't fit under the umbrella. . . . It isn't a serious condition, but it is a life-affecting disability.

Chapter 5

A day in the life of a children's palliative care specialist nurse

Tara Kerr-Elliott and Nicola Eaton

To illustrate how prioritisation occurs in the context of children's palliative care, I have described a specific day from my recent practice. Table 5.1 shows how unexpected situations arose, causing me to reorganise the structure of my day through changing priorities.

On this particular Monday I had planned to go from home, straight to my first planned visit to see a 3-year-old-girl with microcephaly. Whilst her needs are complex and likely to be life-limiting, she has been relatively well and stable for several months prior to a recent hospital admission for prolonged seizures. During this episode she was discharged from hospital with rectal paraldehyde for the treatment of this condition. This morning I planned to train her care worker to administer this new treatment. Our palliative care service incorporates a team of respite care workers, employed by a local voluntary organisation, and my responsibilities include their training and support when providing care to the children on my caseload.

I had planned my morning visits on this occasion based on the location of the children's houses, to keep travelling time to a minimum. I would have started with a visit I was able to do on my way in to work, and then made the other visits, including delivering a blood sample to a hospital, in a geographically logical way.

However, on my way to this visit I received a call from the team administrator, relaying calls from two families on my caseload. The first was from the mother of an 11-year-old with severe junctional epidermolysis bullosa (JEB). His mother was asking if I could visit earlier as he had become unwell over the weekend and had been awake overnight in pain. The second call was from the mother of a 13-year-old in the end-stage of his illness, suffering from a bowel lymphoma. I had met this family the previous week while they were still in hospital. The child was expected to live for a few weeks and we had discussed their options and choices, such as where they would like him to be cared for at the end of his life. They were keen for him to go home and we had agreed that we would aim for discharge from hospital towards the end of this week. His mother had called to say they had actually come home over the weekend and that he was unsettled. His mother had stated that she was not 'too worried' about him but would like a visit at home today.

Table 5.1 A day from practice

Planned day	Actual day
9am: Home visit to 4-year-old-child with microcephaly and complex needs, to train new care worker in the use of rectal paraldehyde	9am: Home visit to 11-year-old child with severe junctional epidermolysis bullosa. Pain reviewed and, after contact with palliative care consultant, symptom advice provided. Blood taken by myself; delivered to hospital by community children's nurse
10:30am: Home visit to 9-year-old child with primary pulmonary hypertension. Routine bloods and central-line dressing required.	11am: Home visit to 13-year-old child with end-stage bowel lymphoma. Child died suddenly but peacefully at 12:15pm: Remained in home, supporting family, contacting professionals at their request. Left at about 4pm.
11:30am: Home visit to 11-year-old child with severe junctional epidermolysis bullosa. Assess symptoms of pain and constipation.	
1–3pm: Office based. Lunch, documentation of visits; work on service's annual report.	
3:30pm: Home visit to 8-year-old child with relapsed Ewing's tumour. Review symptoms and provide support to family.	4pm: Lunch in car, phone calls to team. 4:30pm: Home visit to 8-year-old child with relapsed Ewing's tumour. Analgesia increased after contact with palliative care consultant. Discussion with child's mother about how to answer her child's questions and prepare her siblings for her death.
Plan to finish work at 5pm.	Finished work at 6:15pm.

I realised immediately that both these children required a visit this morning, but I also knew that I would be unable to see them without making alternative arrangements for my other planned visits. There are no other nurses working in the palliative care team but I work closely with the general community children's nursing (CCN) team. I therefore called this team and asked them to see two of the children I had planned to see this morning. Because of staff sickness and their own workload, they were only able to agree to see one. In terms of prioritising on the basis of clinical need, children who are in the end-stages of their illness, or children who have symptoms which are complicated and difficult to manage must always take precedence. A child should never be left uncomfortable or in pain, and it is our aim that families should receive as much support as they need if their wish is for their child to remain at home at the end of his or her life. As the palliative care nurse specialist, I felt these were visits that I should undertake and felt the others were more appropriate for delegation.

As the CCN team could do one of my visits, I asked them to see the child with microcephaly and train her care worker, as this visit was also important, albeit for very different reasons. Because we were now aware that the child required rectal paraldehyde as a rescue treatment for prolonged seizures, her care worker could not safely take sole charge of her without training in the use of the treatment. A delay in providing this training would interrupt the pattern of respite care provided to this child and her family. While it may not be the child's own clinical needs taking priority, the need for parental help in caring for children with complex needs such as these is well-documented, as are the effects on the family of not receiving adequate respite. Within the palliative care service, we focus very much on the needs of the whole family when living with a child with a life-limiting condition, and this focus includes practical, emotional and psychological needs as well as the child's own clinical needs. The mother of this child also has three other children and a disabled, dependent husband. She was already extremely tired following her daughter's recent illness and hospital admission, so I was concerned that any delay in training, resulting in lack of respite care, could have serious implications for this family.

I called the mother of the other child I had planned to see – a 9-year-old with primary pulmonary hypertension. While she is very seriously unwell and awaiting a heart and lung transplant, her condition is relatively stable at this point in time. The visit was to take routine bloods and change the dressing on her central line. These bloods are done monthly and I therefore felt it was acceptable to apologise to the family for cancelling our appointment and rearrange to see her the following day. The alternative option would have been to arrange for her to be seen at her local hospital but, as this should ideally be avoided for any child with a suppressed immune system because of the risk of exposure to hospital-acquired infections, I felt this was an inappropriate and unnecessary risk to take.

I decided to visit the child with JEB first, as his mother had described him as unwell and in pain whereas the mother of the other child had specifically mentioned in her message that she was not 'too worried'. On arrival at the first child's house, I found him looking tired and unwell. I completed a full assessment of his pain and constipation and then called the palliative care consultant, who advised certain medication changes, which I was able to explain to the child and his parents. The child, who is chronically anaemic and blood-transfusion-dependent, was also complaining of symptoms suggesting his anaemia had worsened and I therefore took blood from him, for the CNN team to collect.

I then went to see the second child with a bowel lymphoma. On arrival, I was shocked to find him looking much more unwell than I had anticipated. His breathing was very laboured, he was complaining of pain and he appeared anxious and restless. I assisted his mother in settling him into a comfortable position, and led him through some basic relaxation techniques. After contacting the medical team who had discharged him from hospital, his mother administered some simple oral analgesia. The child settled into a peaceful sleep and died about an hour and a quarter after I had arrived in the home. His death was unexpected in terms of timing but was peaceful and his parents were very pleased that he had been able to die at home, in his own bed and with them by his side. At the family's request I stayed with them until the child's body had been taken to the local chapel of rest. Over the next three hours I was able to provide practical assistance with washing and dressing their son, informing people as they requested, arranging for his death to be certified and contacting the funeral directors of their choice.

I left the family's home about 4 pm, and had a late lunch in my car while making phone calls to my office and the CCN team, whom I asked to obtain and follow-up the blood results from this morning's visit for me. I then went on to my last visit to see an 8-year-old child with a relapsed Ewing's tumour, arriving an hour later than I had arranged.

When reflecting on this particular day in practice, I am able to identify both successful outcomes and those which should lead to a change in my future practice. I believe the most significant mistake I made on this day was not calling back the mothers who had left messages with office staff first thing in the morning. By relying on the team administrator to pass on their messages to me, I believe I wrongly prioritised the order of the visits. If I had spoken to the mother of the dying child personally, I might have been able to establish the urgency of the request for the visit. If I had decided to visit any later, this child might have died in pain. However, while this is my own feeling, his family did not appear to share this view. They expressed only gratitude that I had visited as they had requested (his mother had asked for a visit 'sometime today'). Written feedback from them since his death has confirmed that while the speed of his death had shocked them, they are positive about the peacefulness of his death and feel they were well supported in caring for their son at home, which was where he and they had desperately wanted to be. This feedback can surely be seen as a measure of success in relation to how prioritisation was managed in this instance.

When I visited the child with primary pulmonary hypertension to take her routine blood sample the following day, I was able to apologise to her family in person and provide the care she needed without any compromise to her clinically or, seemingly, to the relationship I have with her and her family. It may be worth noting at this point, however, that, occasionally, fear of recrimination from certain families can wrongly influence decisions taken when prioritising. For example, if a decision arises whereby there is only time to visit one family but two are waiting to be seen, if one family is known to be particularly quick to complain or be aggressive, it can be tempting to prioritise on this basis rather than on the basis of genuine need. I have found that effective and regular clinical supervision, when available, has been a particularly helpful way to deal with these particular issues, with the aim of providing an equitable service recognising equal opportunities based on the needs of children and their families.

I believe that I made the right decision in terms of prioritising visits that I couldn't carry out myself. The child with JEB and the dying child both required specialist symptom care which is within my area of expertise and therefore it was right that I should see these children myself. The care worker training could be, and was, effectively and competently carried out by a CCN, meaning that delegation as a way of prioritising led to respite care being continually provided to a family who were very much in need of it.

At the end of this particular day in practice, while I felt that the children and families had received good care, I arrived home feeling anxious about what I had not had time to do. This did not include the children I had not seen, as I felt I had made appropriate alternative arrangements for them. I was, however, very anxious about my documentation of the day's visits and also about the reports I had planned to do at lunchtime. Though I would always agree that children's clinical needs should take priority, there does seem to be an ever-present tension with important clinical governance issues such as record keeping, auditing and report writing. Looking at my diary for the following day, which now also had an extra visit carried over from today, and also a follow-up visit to the family whose child had died, I realised that I should have time to complete the service's annual report but not the documentation from today's visits. I therefore decided to prioritise this task of record keeping over some of my time off and completed the records at home that evening.

The cases described are not all typical: it is unusual to have to prioritise so dramatically in order to respond to the unexpected death of a child. However, the examples do reflect common dilemmas in terms of having to respond to changing priorities. This description of practice within children's palliative care demonstrates various kinds of prioritisation decisions, influenced by the ultimate aim of providing an effective, equitable service based on clinical need. It also illustrates the impact of having to prioritise on children and their families, the practitioner, other services which are affected by the decisions and those involved in planning and commissioning future services.

Chapter 6

Prioritising paediatric physiotherapy services for children with profound multiple learning difficulties

Elizabeth J. Croot

Background context

This example relates to the provision of physiotherapy for children with profound multiple learning disabilities. The physiotherapists involved were employed by a specialist children's hospital and based in a school for children with profound multiple learning difficulties.

The school had a nursery and admitted children from the age of three on a part-time basis, with the majority attending full time by their fifth birthday. Children left the school at the age of eleven to move to a nearby secondary school. Children below the age of five who were attending the school on a part-time basis were usually seen by the hospital's under-fives physiotherapy service and transferred to the school's service when they reached five years or they started attending school full time, whichever came soonest.

This meant that children would be added to the school physiotherapy caseload throughout the year. The physiotherapy care of children leaving the school at the age of 11 was transferred to the secondary school's physiotherapy team during the summer holidays in the year the child moved schools. As a result the physiotherapy caseload increased throughout the school year. This situation came to a head in a year when the number of children attending the nursery and transferring to the school service far outweighed the number of children due to leave the school.

The situation was compounded when a rotational physiotherapist left the school and was not replaced. The school had minimal input from the occupational therapy service because of staff shortages, and physiotherapy staff were being asked to perform certain functions that had previously been the responsibility of an occupational therapist. The increasing caseload and the decrease in staffing meant that it was impossible to provide optimal levels of care to all children at the school. This caused a dilemma because of the different needs of the children at all stages in their school careers.

Younger children were transferred from the under-fives service, where they had received one-to-one therapy with a parent or carer present, into a school where parents were not necessarily present during treatment. The school therapists had to get to know the children and to build relationships with their parents. Parents often required support and reassurance at this transition time. Many were concerned that they would not have the same access to a physiotherapist and that their children would not receive the same high standard of service at school as they had received from the under-fives service.

Younger children have more potential for motor development because of their age. Treatment is aimed at improving their abilities and preventing deformities that would limit their abilities and cause discomfort and pain in later life. They require active-therapy treatment towards developmental goals as well as provision of equipment and orthotics. In addition, school staff are unfamiliar with the children and need advice about handling them, and guidance towards suitable activities for them.

Several of the older children at the school had developed deformities in spite of attempts to prevent these. Children with deformities need treatment and equipment to correct or accommodate these in order to delay the progression of these deformities and the need for surgical correction. Many of these children did go on to have surgical interventions at some stage and they needed intensive physiotherapy, with advice and support to parents and school staff following surgery.

Prioritisation action

Having identified the need to prioritise the caseload, staff met with the service manager to discuss how this could be achieved. In this meeting the physiotherapists working at the special school identified factors which influenced decisions about which children to prioritise.

Factors identified were:

- the age of the child
- type and severity of movement disorder
- co-existing morbidity e.g. visual or hearing difficulties
- prognosis
- therapist time available
- level of parental involvement
- concurrent interventions e.g. surgery, botullinum toxin injections.

Following this meeting a literature search was carried out to locate evidence to inform decisions about how to prioritise physiotherapy treatment for children with profound multiple learning disabilities. Findings from this search were discussed in relation to the context of the special school physiotherapy service within the school, the wider physiotherapy service and the multidisciplinary team.

It was decided that physiotherapy aims and interventions should be delivered in one of two ways:

1   Postural management – this meant providing a positioning programme (24-hour where necessary) using a range of orthoses and positioning equipment

as required. The aim of this approach was to prevent, correct or accommodate deformity as appropriate, provide a variety of positions for the individual and to enable the individual to participate in activities at home and at school. This intervention would be implemented and reviewed at appropriate intervals depending on the individual child.

2   Active intervention – this meant providing more intensive bursts of active treatment for children in special circumstances e.g. post-surgery. This intervention was targeted towards specific goals for the child and was time limited. Following a period of active intervention, the child's postural management programme would be reviewed and revised if necessary, and the child would revert to a postural management programme.

These options for service provision were underpinned by a commitment to provide an integrated service, taking into account the needs of the child, the family and carers, and school staff in developing appropriate advice and support. The rationale for this was based on the evidence that was found to support different methods and approaches to treatment. For example, the use of postural management programmes was supported by evidence that:

- maintaining symmetry with correct positioning reduces the risk of deformity
- postural management equipment provides proximal stabilisation from which to facilitate active, controlled and functional movement
- positioning equipment allows the child to experience a number of different positions and contributes to the sensory, psychological, intellectual and social development of the child.

(Pountney et al. 1990, 1999, 2002; Kalen and Bleck 1985)

Evaluation

Evaluation of the changes in practice has been conducted through on-going reflection on the impact of the changes made.

Immediately after deciding these changes, physiotherapy staff felt more confident about answering school staff and parents' enquiries about discrepancies in the amount of treatment received by different children. Physiotherapists felt more in control of the caseload and experienced reduced stress in relation to caseload pressures.

The change to intensive periods of treatment facilitated focused and goal-directed treatment to a greater extent than continuous and ongoing treatment. As a result, physiotherapists spent more time assessing and goal setting than had previously been the case. This led to more frequent communication between physiotherapists, parents and school staff as assessment findings were discussed and goals negotiated and set.

There were difficulties in identifying criteria to determine the optimal times for children to receive intensive periods of treatment. There were also discussions about whether these periods should be time limited or dependent on the child achieving the goals set for the period. These discussions are ongoing.

School staff found the disruption to the child's timetable easier to manage as the timings for intensive periods of treatment were negotiated and planned in advance where possible. Despite this, periods of active treatment were interrupted at times by unforeseen circumstances, for example, changes in the child's health or home or school situation.

The need for flexibility within the system remained, and physiotherapists continued to respond immediately to significant changes in a child's ability, equipment, school or home circumstances, regardless of whether that child was currently receiving active treatment. Unforeseen changes often led to a period of treatment becoming necessary in order for the child to return to a postural management programme.

The integrated approach to postural management meant that if one aspect of the programme changed, other components had to be revised to accommodate the change. For example, a child beginning to use a spinal jacket would require a review of their standing and seating equipment.

There were cost implications with the introduction of comprehensive postural management programmes where a wider range of equipment and orthotics were required by the children than previously. These costs should eventually be offset by a reduction in the amount of surgery needed.

There have been opportunities for physiotherapy staff to develop and refine their practice within the original framework of treatment. Examples of this include work to develop and implement more comprehensive postural management programmes utilising the latest developments in orthotics and equipment, and an investigation and trial of different therapy outcome measures designed for use with this patient group.

Implementation of this framework of treatment has highlighted some of the tensions inherent in delivering a child-centred service where the needs of parents, carers and school staff must also be taken into account. Clearly physiotherapists have to balance the needs, abilities and limitations of all parties in determining how and when to intervene. The work described in this example has been a catalyst for further discussions about some of the constraints to clinical decision making in this situation and problem-solving approaches to overcome these.

The author wishes to acknowledge the contribution of David Threlfall and Pauline Gladwin to the work described above.

References

Kalen, V. and Bleck, E. E. (1985) 'Prevention of spastic paraplegic dislocation of the hip', *Developmental Medicine and Child Neurology*, **27**: 17–24.

Poutney, T. E., Mulcahy, C. M. and Green, E. M. (1990) 'Early development of postural control', *Physiotherapy*, **76**: 799–802.

Poutney, T. E., Green, E. M., Mulcahy, C. M. and Nelham, R. L. (1999) 'The Chailey approach to postural managment', *Association of Paediatric Chartered Physiotherapists Journal*, March, 15–33.

Poutney, T.E., Mandy, A., Green, E.M. and Gard, P. (2002) 'Management of hip dislocation with postural management', *Child: Care Health and Development*, **28**(2) 179–85.

Chapter 7

Triage in speech and language therapy

Caroline Pickstone

Background context

Speech and language delay is one of the commonest reasons for concern amongst parents of preschool children, and a survey of speech and language therapy (SLT) contact data shows that children take up 56 per cent of the total available provision (van der Gaag *et al.*, 1999). Not surprisingly, the demand for SLT resources outstrips their supply and service managers have had to be creative in using resources efficiently and effectively. Historically, waiting lists for SLT have tended to be long in many areas of the UK, potentially resulting in long waits for children with urgent needs. Although the impact of waiting lists for parents and children can only be surmised, it may potentially affect their relationship with therapists where parents are highly anxious or make a complaint. It seems that waiting for therapy may be very stressful for parents and causes concern to practitioners and managers.

How then can the demand be managed? This chapter reviews a local approach to caseload management and examines the learning and the impact of changes in services for children now and in the future. The work began in the early 1990s and was a response to long waiting lists for assessment and intervention for children. Having previously been organised in departments serving sectors of a city, SLT practitioners were brought together as one service covering the whole city. Waiting lists for therapy were evident in all sectors but varied across the city, averaging 12 months' waiting overall. Small teams of therapists had operated autonomously, holding their own waiting lists for assessment and for intervention, which had allowed marked differences to arise across the city. Managers suspected that there was considerable inequity in therapy provision using this system and felt that they needed a change of approach which would provide them with more information about the needs of children waiting for therapy and staffing required. Given the very high demand, reducing lost clinical time was essential. There was growing recognition that services needed to meet local needs and be offered in accessible settings. Triage was the approach chosen to manage waiting for assessment and therapy. It relies on three main elements: triage appointments, prioritisation, and active caseload management by teams of staff.

Triage appointments

The process of triage is shown in Figure 7.1. Incoming referrals were checked by team leaders, who maintained an overview of the numbers and nature of referrals and picked up on any errors, duplications or additional needs (including inter-preters). Appointments were offered with a small number of experienced therapists (four) to try to maximise consistency in terms of decision making. Their experience ranged from 9 to 26 years.

Although many features of this first contact with a family will be familiar to practitioners, there were some distinctive aspects in the local application. First, following referral, parents were contacted by letter and asked to phone a central number to book an appointment. The advantage of encouraging parents to initiate the contact and centralising the booking was that parents could then choose a clinic

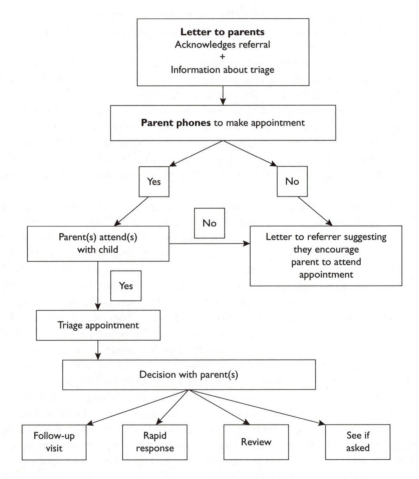

Figure 7.1 The triage process

and a time that was convenient from the full range of options including short-notice cancellations. A local audit revealed that 85 per cent of parents responded to the letter asking them to make contact. The effect on attendance was dramatic and parents who booked appointments attended triage clinics, reducing time wasted. A centralised system allowed managers to monitor and plan the numbers of clinics needed. It also appeared that parents who were highly concerned tended to make contact as soon as the letter was received, resulting in earlier appointments.

Second, the triage appointment was designed to allow parents to meet an experienced therapist who could discuss their concerns and gather initial background information. It allowed the therapist to observe the parent and child using a two-way mirror and to reach a decision with the parent and child about whether they needed to take any action at the time. The observation of parent–child interaction was valuable in many ways, allowing the therapist to observe the child in a relaxed interaction with a familiar adult and providing a rapid insight into expressive language and play. The majority of children settled easily and engaged with the parent readily, given a range of familiar toy materials. Many parents reported that they were reassured by this and felt that the therapist had seen a representative example of their child's skills on which to base decisions about immediate management. The triage therapist made a decision with the parent based on whether the child needed to be seen again and if so, on the urgency of the need.

When the family did not contact to make the initial triage appointment or did not attend, the letter to the referrer informed them of this and suggested that they might wish to encourage the family to make contact. Where this was not possible, therapists tried to work to identify another carer who was able to work with the child if intervention was required.

Prioritisation

Prioritisation was the second element in triage and the decision related to the *initial* course of management for a child. This decision used a prioritisation system based on the work of Ward *et al.* (1990). The approach identified factors to be considered in making decisions about intervention and recognised the potential for spontaneous recovery within 6 months of the appointment. Factors taken into account included the age of the child, the nature of their difficulty, the level of parental concern and anxiety, the likely effectiveness of intervention, the urgency (were other actions contingent on the results of intervention, e.g. reports for special educational needs process), the anticipated level of parental involvement, whether there was a risk of problems worsening and whether timing was optimum.

Aspects of the implementation did arouse some resistance by practitioners, usually because of misunderstandings about triage as a method. Some of those misunderstandings may usefully be addressed here:

• Triage does not replace diagnostic assessment; a full assessment would be offered as a rapid response package if necessary.

- Rapid response packages consisted of six weekly sessions to start management through diagnostic assessment and intervention; it was never the intention that six sessions would be the sum total of intervention offered but rather would provide an initial intervention.
- At triage, therapists asked parents for their views about the referral and possible intervention and checked whether they would prefer to wait and see whether the child progressed without help, recognising that parents and therapists may have different views about whether therapy is timely or indicated (Glogowska and Campbell, 2000; Marshall *et al.*, 2004). Parents or carers were free to refer back at any time.
- Finally, triage did not eliminate waiting altogether, despite careful allocation of time and planning. There may be a wait for intervention but parents knew how long that wait was likely to be.

Active caseload management

The third element in successful local implementation of triage was caseload management as a team rather than by individuals. Therapists were concerned about the length of the waiting lists in the city and were keen to manage these, but the move to centralised caseloads was a major change. Any change process presents challenges and requires clarity of vision and sustained effort. Although there have been some changes latterly, staff worked in teams and met regularly to review and allocate the workload for the next 12 weeks. This allocation and planning was directed by experienced team leaders who also carried out the triage appointments and therefore had a current overview of the needs of children waiting for intervention. Part of the team leader's role was to allocate the team's workload to allow sufficient time to be set aside for nursery and home visits, rapid-response appointments and reviews. This time allocation remains essential if the timescales for rapid response are to be achieved.

Evaluation

The implementation of triage led to reductions in the wait for first appointments and therapy intervention which have been sustained. It offered a way of making decisions about children referred for SLT to determine their level of priority for therapy, allowing a reduction in waiting time for those who are likely to derive the greatest benefit. Reflecting on the early evolution of triage, it is possible to make several observations about the implementation. First, referral agents were not required to make any real changes to the way that they worked, but information about the rationale for triage and the likely impact on waiting lists would have been useful. In fact, it took some time before the service was able to shake off the reputation amongst some health visitors for long waiting lists, even when the new system was running smoothly, and this may have impacted on the number of referrals (Keating *et al.*, 1998). Second, there was an impact on other services and resources. Given that language difficulties and hearing problems may co-occur, changes to the speed of response of SLT services may have knock-on effects for others such as audiology. The need for observation facilities in order to run triage most successfully has implications in terms of planning for accommodation in the long term. One of the main pillars for successful triage is good IT systems to support central booking and information for practitioners. It seems that because the approach evolved in response to waiting lists rather than being a planned implementation of a proven approach, some of the strategic planning did not take place; the effects of this lack of multi-professional planning have been revealed over time. Finally, there was no systematic approach to gaining user views on triage, which would have enhanced our understanding of parent and child perspectives on this approach.

Children's services in the UK are changing (DfES 2003; DoH 2003) and the question arises of whether triage is relevant now. The present healthcare agenda emphasises access and inclusion for disadvantaged groups and encourages user involvement to shape high quality provisions. Triage is now cited as being good practice (Hall and Elliman 2003) but further development has been undertaken locally to dovetail triage with models of SLT involvement in Sure Start and other community-based programmes. In the context of such programmes, the issues surrounding parental anxiety and potential for involvement in therapy need to be considered. Although 85 per cent of parents who were referred contacted SLT to make an appointment, we know little about the remaining 15 per cent who did not do so. As with other 'screening' approaches, some parents will respond to a further prompt to contact whereas others will be hard to reach and require alternative approaches (Grunfeld 1997). It seems reasonable to assume that a considerable proportion of those who did not make contact are disadvantaged and therefore eligible for Sure Start services. The prioritisation decision based on Ward's system gives higher priority to parents who are anxious and to those who may be expected to take an active part in intervention. Some parents may not have a clear idea of what to expect in terms of developmental progress and this could impact on their level of anxiety (Anon 1997). Some will not be able to take part in interventions because of other factors in their life at the time. The risk is that children will be precluded from intervention because of difficulties in securing a parent or carer to work with them to implement a programme. Practitioners face this problem regularly and are creative in establishing ways of maximising the effectiveness of intervention by working with staff in day care and other early years settings.

The nature of triage will reflect the role of SLT practitioners in community settings with targeted populations at risk for language problems. If they use flexible approaches, including home visiting or drop-in sessions as a first point of contact with families whose children are at risk, this will affect what is needed for children referred for triage. Many speech and language therapists in early childhood pro-grammes like Sure Start do not carry a caseload but may be involved with at-risk children in groups or by means of their support for outreach workers. If the child has long-term language needs, triage will be their point of entry to the SLT service.

Careful liaison between Sure Start services and the triage therapists is likely to encourage attendance, minimise parents' anxiety and ensure a smooth transition. Triage sessions that combine local hearing tests with speech and language assessment have been welcomed because they reduce the number of appointments and streamline decision making by having results available to the therapist immediately. In this way, triage remains valid in the current climate, and flexible application of triage continues to offer an approach which is transparent in addressing the question of whether therapy intervention is needed.

References

Anon (1997) *Key findings from a nationwide survey among parents of zero to three year olds*. Chicago: Zero to Three. Accessed 28 May 2005 at www.zerotothree.org/parent _poll.html-8k

DfES (2003) *Every Child Matters. Cm 5860*. London: The Stationery Office.

DoH (2003) *Getting the Right Start: National Service Framework for Children, Emerging Findings*. London: Department of Health.

Glogowska, M. and Campbell, R. (2000) 'Investigating parental views of involvement in preschool speech and language therapy', *International Journal of Language and Communication Disorders*, **35**: 391–406.

Grunfeld, E. (1997) 'Cervical cancer; screening hard to reach groups', *Canadian Medical Association Journal*, **157**: 543–5.

Hall, D. M. B. and Elliman, D. (2003) *Health for all children*. Oxford: Oxford University Press.

Keating, D., Syrmis, M., Hamilton, L. and McMahon, S. (1998) 'Paediatricians: Referral rates and speech pathology waiting lists', *Journal of Paediatric Child Health*, **34**: 451–5.

Marshall, J., Phillips, J. and Goldbart, J. (2004) 'He's just lazy, he'll do it when he goes to school.' Parents and speech and language therapists' explanatory models of language delay. A paper presented to the Health R&D North West Annual Research Conference. June 2004.

Van Der Gaag, A., McLoone, P. and Reid, D. (1999) 'Speech and language therapy caseloads in seven districts in the UK', *Journal of Management in Medicine*, **13**: 23–32.

Ward, S., Birkett, D. and Kellett, B. (1990) 'An expert way of prioritising clients', *Speech Therapy in Practice*, **5**.

Chapter 8

The least first framework

Rosemarie Hayhow

This example of a framework to assist prioritisation was developed for young children who stammer or stutter. It originated as a way of organising the different treatment options in a training course for speech and language therapists (SLTs) rather than from a need to consider caseload management. However, several therapists saw the relevance of the training model to their clinical decision making and so the framework was developed

Background context

Stuttering is a low incidence problem and so many SLTs have little experience with this client group, leading to anxiety and low levels of confidence. Less experienced SLTs need to be clear about the boundaries of their competence and their role with this client group. SLTs learn direct and indirect treatment approaches in training at pre-qualification and postgraduate levels but may not see these put into practice.

The two most widely used indirect approaches are parent–child interaction therapy, which was developed by Rustin and colleagues (Rustin *et al.* 1996) and the demands : capacities (D:C) model (see Stewart and Turnbull 1995 for a full description). Both aim to alter the communication environment so as to maximise the chances of the child developing normal fluency skills. Parents may be advised to become more child-centred in their communication style by choosing topics that are immediately relevant to the child's interests and current activities and by asking fewer adult-orientated questions. Adult rate of speech, speed of responding or turn taking patterns within the family may also be modified. Children's speech and language skills may be assessed and considered in relation to the demands made of the child in communication and general behaviour. Both approaches can be used without children being aware that their stuttering is targeted, although work on fluency skills could be a part of D:C therapy. The approaches feel safe, as there is no direct attention on the child's speaking or stuttering; it is the parents who make the changes.

Direct therapy involves working directly on the child's stuttering with the full knowledge of the child. In this country, the Lidcombe program (Onslow *et al.* 2002)

is becoming the most widely used direct approach. It is a behavioural programme that requires weekly clinic sessions to teach parents how to respond to children's stutter-free and stuttered speech.

Decisions regarding the need for therapy are complicated by the high rate of natural recovery in early stuttering and the knowledge that severity of stuttering at onset is not a prognostic indicator (Yairi and Ambrose 1999). The clinician must therefore weigh up the factors that put children at risk for persistent stuttering and offset these against low-risk factors that would suggest a transient problem.

There is also anxiety that inappropriate management could make stuttering worse. The idea that awareness of stuttering may increase the severity stems from Johnson's work published in 1955 with his suggestion that parents' negative evaluations of the child's developmental disfluencies leads to stuttering. Although there is no evidence to support his claims, the anxiety lives on, perhaps because we still have no agreed explanation of what causes and maintains early stuttering.

The timing of treatment is also important: there is consensus that, with increasing age, stuttering tends to become more severe and also increasingly difficult to treat. There is also an increased risk of relapse after treatment. The longer the stuttering lasts, the greater the risk that the child will suffer emotional, social or psychological damage. But caution is needed if we are to avoid pathologising a transient phenomenon or wasting resources on something that will resolve naturally. So the questions for the clinician are: Does this child need treatment of some sort? If so, what sort of treatment might be appropriate? Who is the best person to provide it?

Prioritisation action

The framework to assist decision making was called the 'least first framework' in recognition that resources should not be wasted, natural recovery should be given a fair chance and therapists should be wary of becoming part of the attempted solutions that maintain the problem (Fisch *et al.* 1982). To clarify the options available to SLTs, these are separated into three levels showing the assessment areas and indicators that help decide upon action. This framework is not meant to be a set of rules but rather should be viewed as a kind of map to guide SLTs while they keep in mind the principle of doing as little as necessary. When therapists lack confidence with young children who stutter, they may want to do as little as *possible* but this is very different from as little as *necessary*. They need to feel skilful up to the level at which they intervene and to be clear about when to refer on for more specialist help. Since we cannot predict with certainty what will happen to the stuttering of these young children, SLTs need to be clear that they should formulate a hypothesis. They can then monitor the effects of their intervention decision to see if their hypothesis was correct.

Some services favour early discharge if no therapy is being offered. I would argue against this because of the unpredictability of early stuttering. Individual therapists need to know whether their hypotheses were correct if they are to learn from their experiences with these children. Also an SLT service can only monitor the effectiveness of its procedures by knowing the individual outcomes in the longer term. Additionally, parents may think, for example, that assessment and information is all that the service has to offer if they are discharged without some form of follow-up. They may not then seek re-referral when the stuttering fails to resolve or returns at a later date. It is not unusual to see an older child who is stuttering quite severely who was originally seen before school and whose parents thought there was nothing more the service could offer. If the therapist is clear about the structure of the service then this can be explained to parents, thus avoiding any misunderstandings about what is available.

The framework

The least first framework is summarised in Table 8.1.

Level one is the simplest in terms of assessment and intervention as the child will present as relatively low risk for persistent stuttering. Assessment will include a full history of the stuttering and observations of both the child's and parents' communication skills in an informal context. Relevant background information will be discussed and the parental concerns, knowledge about stuttering and current strategies explored. Intervention is focused on providing information and negotiating a management plan that will include some monitoring of the child's stuttering.

Level two may follow on from level one if the stuttering doesn't resolve or if the child seems at risk for persistent stuttering at referral. For example, there may be a family history of persistent stuttering or the child may have been stuttering for more than six months. Intervention will include information and negotiation as in level one, and specific strategies may be put in place to reduce demands on communication or develop the child's capacities. Some regular clinical contact will be required to monitor the effects of the strategies and to ensure that they are being used as intended.

Level three may follow on from level one or two if the stuttering doesn't resolve or may be the first choice if the child presents as a high risk for persistent stuttering at referral. There is usually a longer history of stuttering for a potential level-three child, more to discuss about management so far, and the effects of this and the effects of the stuttering on both child and family. At this level a specialist therapist will be involved, either in delivering the direct therapy or by being available for supervision of less experienced colleagues.

The local context will influence the exact interpretation of these levels and the circumstances in which direct or indirect therapy will be offered. Levels should be reviewed regularly in the light of new research evidence and reappraised with reference to referral patterns and longer-term outcomes for this client group. Services vary in terms of the balance of resources they offer at levels one, two and three depending upon their preferences and the levels of expertise available for direct versus indirect approaches. A recent study by Franken *et al.* (2005) suggests

Level	Indicators	Assessment	Intervention
One	Early referral, i.e close to onset Episodic, apparently getting better Current parental strategies helpful Evidence of self correction No family history or history of recovery No awareness Little parental concern	Clear description of fluency problem Date and nature of onset Description of stammering behaviour and % syllables stuttered Factors that influence severity Episodic vs consistent Changes since onset Family history Parental intervention and effect Relevant background information Informal assessment of: • speech and language • parent–child interaction • general development	Provide information Devise strategies rather than give advice Monitor changes: keep diary, speech ratings Active review: phone or clinic visit, timescale, decision factors
Two	Referral >6 months after onset Parents feel need for help and are keen to be involved Child becoming aware of stammering Increasing frequency and severity of stammering Less episodic Parent resistant to direct therapy, or regular clinic visits not possible Level one limited/short-term effect	As level one if new referral Effects of level-one intervention if appropriate Child's readiness for direct therapy Parents' resources and wishes Formulation of hypotheses	Problem solving with parent(s) to help develop fluency Changes in parental communication Reduction in demands Increase in child's capacities Process to monitor effect of intervention Reformulation of hypotheses if necessary

Three	Child stuttering for >1 year Environment supportive: general and communication Child distressed, stammering having negative effect Family history of persistent stammering Parents keen to 'work' with child Child responsive to adult-led activities Levels one and two have been tried	Levels one and two as relevant Child's awareness of stammering Child/parents' level of concern Description of pattern of stammering since onset	Direct therapy, e.g. Lidcombe program Possibly work with school Remember, with increasing age, parental influence on communication environment is lessened and generalisation of clinic or home fluency may be more problematic. It is not in the child's best interest to delay direct therapy

Figure 8.1 The least first framework

that it is feasible to compare indirect methods with the more researched direct methods like the Lidcombe program (Jones *et al*. 2005). But we are a long way from being able to make informed choices regarding the best therapy options for individual children.

The process

At referral there may be information to indicate the most likely level of intervention and so at this point the child could be assigned to a generalist who will monitor natural recovery or to a specialist who will start therapy. Referral descriptions suggestive of the different levels might be:

> *Level one*: 'This child has been stuttering for the last two months, there is no family history of stuttering and the parents would like some advice'.
>
> *Level two*: 'This child started to stutter severely five months ago, it seems to be getting better but the parents would like some advice on how to deal with the stuttering at home.'
>
> *Level three*: 'This child has been stuttering for over a year and the parents are concerned as it seems to be getting worse. The child was reluctant to speak to me when I visited the home so I can't describe the stuttering but I can verify that the mother is a reliable informant.'

SLTs, with the support of the British Stammering Association (1999), have encouraged health professionals to refer early so that appropriate monitoring can be put in place. Early direct treatment may not always suit parent and child. It is therefore reassuring that children's progress with the Lidcome program is not compromised when they start therapy at age four rather than closer to onset (Kingston *et al*. 2003). There may be advantages in waiting a while before starting direct treatment, but care needs to be taken that parents do not exhaust their energy and commitment in other treatments before starting the Lidcombe program. The idea that there may be an optimal timeframe to start a course of direct and somewhat demanding parent-based therapy is tantalising. With a framework such as the least first framework, the idea of timing is relevant, although decisions regarding optimal timing will be reached through discussion rather than by reference to the literature since there is, as yet, no conclusive indicative evidence. The following factors may be relevant to the timing of level three interventions:

- family ability to incorporate the rigours of treatment into family life
- extent of the child's distress
- extent of the parents' distress
- the severity of the stuttering – frequency and severity
- a pattern of increasing severity since onset
- the extent that stuttering impedes communication
- parental attempts to help with stuttering, effect of these

- ease with which parents give specific feedback on their child's behaviour
- parents' ability to organise activities with their child and the child's responsiveness to this.

This is not a definitive list but rather indicates the areas that can be discussed when weighing up whether this is the right time for the child and the parents.

Evaluation

The model has helped some services develop care pathways for a child who stammers or stutters, identify training needs within a department and facilitated the development of specialist skills and posts. Some problems have been encountered when the framework has been interpreted in a hierarchical manner with each level being worked through. These are not steps to be completed but levels to help therapists and parents make the best decisions at a particular time, with a clear idea of what might follow if initial hypotheses are proved incorrect. The framework can be used by SLTs who have sole responsibility for all stuttering referrals, as well as to help structure a service. At a more abstract level, the framework is content free and so has the potential to be used with new treatment options as they become available. However, like all frameworks, it should be subjected to regular scrutiny and overhauled to ensure that it continues to represent a workable and useful way of looking at stuttering and intervention options. In my own clinical work I use levels one and three. Level two is included in recognition of the clinical justifications for the indirect approaches.

References

British Stammering Association (1999) *Primary healthcare workers project* available on their website www.stammering.org

Fisch, R., Weakland, J. and Segal, L. (1982) *The tactics of change: doing therapy briefly.* California: Jossey-Bass.

Franken, M-C., Kielstra-Van der Schalk, C. and Boelens, H. (2005) 'Experimental treatment of early stuttering: A preliminary study', *Journal of Fluency Disorders*, **30**: 189–99.

Johnson, W. (ed.) (1955) *Stuttering in children and adults.* Minneapolis: University of Minnesota Press.

Jones, M., Onslow, M., Packman, A., Williams, S., Ormond, T., Schwarz, T. and Gebski, V. (2005) 'A randomised controlled trial of the Lidcombe program for early stuttering intervention', *British Medical Journal*, **331**: 659–61.

Kingston, M., Huber, A., Onslow, M., Jones, M. and Packman, A. (2003) 'Predicting treatment time with the Lidcombe Program: Replication and meta-analysis'. *International Journal of Language and Communication Disorders*, **38**: 165–177.

Onslow, M., Packman, A. and Harrison,E. (2002) *The Lidcombe Program of early stuttering intervention: A clinician's guide.* Austin, Texas: Pro-ed publishers.

Rustin, L., Botterill, W. and Kelman, E. (1996) *Assessment and therapy for young disfluent children: family interaction.* London: Whurr.

Stewart, T. and Turnbull, J. (1995) *Working with Dysfluent Children*. Bicester: Winslow Press.

Yairi, E. and Ambrose, N. G. (1999) 'Early childhood stuttering I: Persistency and recovery rates', *Journal of Speech, Language and Hearing Research*, **42**: 1097–112

Part III

Perspectives from theory

Chapter 9

Thinking

Where to start

Michael Loughlin

A modest goal

The actor and Quaker Paul Eddington once said that if you can get through life without actually seriously harming anyone then you are doing all right, and consequently his modest goal in life was to leave the Earth in no worse a state than he had found it. This, he observed, is rather more difficult than it might at first seem, and anyone who thinks otherwise has probably failed to appreciate the number of ways in which one's life affects the lives of others.

This straightforward claim has since been labelled the Principle of Non-Maleficence by authors in the field of bioethics (Beauchamp and Childress 2001) who have devoted many pages of text to discussing various 'formulations' of the 'principle' and its alleged relationship with other supposedly foundational principles. So many, in fact, and so many of them printed on non-recycled paper, that they have almost certainly contributed to our current ecological crisis, thereby violating the principle and proving Eddington's point in the process. Despite its unfortunate association with such unhelpful academic exercises, Eddington's 'modest goal' still strikes me as worth pursuing, though as a beneficiary of an economic system that condemns at least 2000 children[1] per day to utterly pointless deaths from poverty-related disease and malnutrition, I suspect I have pursued it with only very limited success at best.

For this reason I was reluctant to contribute an 'ethical' component to a book about how practitioners working with children make prioritising decisions, especially when the editor explained to me that I would be expected to comment on real examples of practitioners struggling to do the right thing under difficult circumstances. As a student of 'applied philosophy', I am frequently struck by the pernicious influence that theorists of all sorts, philosophers included, have had on debates about how practices should be conducted in the areas of health, education, social policy and in organisations generally. I have argued that, as theorists, we need to think more carefully about the ways in which we comment on such practices, and to realise not only that our work may do no positive good, but that it may even actually be harmful (Loughlin 2002a, b, 2004a, b, c). Attempts to 'apply' academic perspectives to practice tend too often to fall into either one of two simplistic approaches, each corresponding to an unhelpful and largely parasitic social role.

On the one hand there is the academic as 'the Boss's Helper'. This academic works for government and/or senior management, producing policy documents to help evaluate and regulate practices in a given area (Loughlin 2002a, 2004a). Whatever the stated parameters of the role and whatever the academic's sincere intention, the *de facto* role of such work is to find new ways for the powers that be to tell the workforce that they are rubbish. Since the unexciting conclusion that people are generally doing as well as can reasonably be expected (but maybe they could do even better if they were better resourced, better supported, better paid and had more time off) is unlikely to strike those officials who commissioned the work as a very substantial outcome, the authors of commissioned work are under pressure to recommend some manner of change in workers' practices. Any serious contributor to this 'applied research' culture (meaning, anyone who wants their recommendations to be taken seriously by those who control the sources of funding) knows that 'reform' must always precede investment. So, all too often, such research is the cue for reorganisation exercises, costly not only in financial terms but in staff time and morale. The need to ensure that the changes are made provides the rationale for a culture of perpetual monitoring, creating new layers of management and the diversion of yet more resources from the front-line workforce.

On the other hand, there is the academic as 'Self-Help Therapist'. This sort of academic purports to offer guidance in the form of general principles and/or theoretical models which, if thoroughly internalised by individual practitioners, will make them better at whatever it is they do (Loughlin 2002b, 2004b, c). The improvements on offer range from the ability to harness their natural capacities and develop more effective 'leadership skills' (Moss 2003) to the ability to 'cultivate moral excellence' (Kottow 2004). Whatever the author's stated intention, the *de facto* role of such work is to find new ways for members of the workforce to tell *themselves* that they are rubbish, and then to supply them with spurious mantras to make them feel better about it – to reassure them that, just by reading the published work, they are at least doing something about their general ignorance, lack of generic skills, lack of ethical awareness and lack of reflexivity. The advice offered is rarely very specific. Nor, stripped of jargon, is it typically particularly insightful.[2] As David Seedhouse puts it in a brutally honest assessment, such theorists usually 'have nothing more to say than any reasonably educated person could come up with, given a few days off work' (Seedhouse 1996).

In each case the outcome is the same. Practitioners are either coerced or seduced into re-describing and evaluating their practices in terms of a new and alien language, one that in no way evolved from the context of their daily work. Though no clear demonstration is ever given that this re-description actually improves practices, the new language becomes trendy in a given area and learning its key phrases becomes essential if one wants to 'get on', to impress one's managers and perhaps even one's peers, or at least to avoid being seen as conservative, complacent, dogmatic, unreflective, behind the times or just plain unethical. In most contemporary organisations, just about the worst sin one can be accused of is being 'resistant to change': so the insistence (characteristic of any genuinely professional outlook) that one is provided with good evidence that change is for the better *before* one 'embraces' it, is interpreted as symptomatic of some moral or psychological flaw. Since the processes of theoretical innovation are ongoing in the age of 'life-long learning', this means that we can look forward to a future in professional life of continuously learning new sets of guidelines and regulatory frameworks, associated with new models and mantras, only for that 'new knowledge' to become out of date almost as soon as we have become accustomed to it.

Even if many practitioners say they actually want this sort of 'assistance', it does not follow that as intellectuals we ought to provide it. To proceed as though this does follow is to make all manner of assumptions about the relationship between expressed wants, need and benefit that any credible academic should recognise as at least highly contentious, and so not the sort of thing one may legitimately simply assume. Contrary to some of the more simplistic proponents of classical economics, most mature human beings recognise that they do not always want what is best for them, nor is the fact that certain wants are expressed in certain contexts evidence that people really want, let alone need, the thing they say that they want in that context – for what they may need most is for the context to change. Certainly, what most public sector workers want seems to me (speaking for the moment simply as a public sector worker) to be the sort of thing we are not supposed to mention in any debate about 'prioritising': more resources, more support, more money and more time off.

Such concerns are ruled out in any debate about 'prioritising' because the whole point of such a debate is not to complain that one has not got enough resources, but to think rationally about how to make the best use of the resources one has. The debate takes it as read that one lacks the resources to do all one wants. Since that is, however regrettably, 'the reality', any 'rational' professional will realise there is no point moaning about it and will want instead to think about how to prioritise the resources available. The focus cannot be on what is wrong with the context that necessitates prioritising, because by definition that is not what the debate is about. Indeed, if you tell professionals to say what they want and/or need in a 'realistic' context – meaning, precisely, one in which all of the above good things (more resources etc.) are not available – then they may well reply that they want or need advice on how to prioritise the limited resources they have. Any academic who hopes to be 'useful' to the professional will therefore try to help him or her find some determinate answer to *that* question. In contrast, an academic who suggests that the context may be such that it renders a rational, determinate answer to that question impossible has thereby failed to say anything 'useful'.

And here is where I can stop speaking simply as a public sector worker and begin to speak, also, as a philosopher. Not because as a philosopher I have some special insight about prioritising that others lack. Certainly not because, as a philosopher, I somehow know how to prioritise care for children better than people who work with children on a daily basis. Rather it is because one thing philosophy teaches you to question, consistently, is how debates get framed: why some things are ruled out of the context of a debate from the outset, while other things get labelled the really 'practical' concerns – the truly important business of the day. Nothing is useful (or useless) *per se*; things are useful or useless given certain assumptions, interests and agendas. Debates are framed with reference to a background of such assumptions, interests and agendas. It is because of the way the prioritising debate is framed that most academics who contribute to it fall into the role of either The Boss's Helper or The Self-Help Therapist, or in the worst cases straddle both roles. Yet academics, of all people, should be willing and able to ask the questions: what is the purpose of my activity? Whose agendas am I serving? Which assumptions and interests frame this debate, and do I want to endorse them implicitly by naively contributing to it?

Why, then, despite my misgivings, did I agree to contribute to a book called 'Prioritising child health: practice and principles'? It was because the editor assured me that I could use my contribution to attempt to shift the focus of the debate – to write not about 'how to prioritise', not to join in the quest for 'principles' that will determine good practice in prioritising healthcare for children, since it is by no means clear that I have the appropriate knowledge to comment on this. Rather, the editor offered me the chance to comment on the role, meaning and limitations of this quest: why should we be looking for principles in the first place? Why should we assume that a person who can find no such principles (beyond banalities – points that everyone, whatever their academic background, could agree to) has somehow 'failed'? What reason is there to believe that practitioners who know of no such principles are practising badly, or ineffectively, or somehow not as well as they might do? On the basis of which claims – about (for instance) rationality and about what it means to do well in a given context – might such a belief be justified?

Obviously, wherever we work, if we care about what we do then we will want to think carefully about how to do it as well as possible, but that banal observation implies no specific conclusion about the best way for any given group of workers to go about the task, nor does it imply anything about the limitations of that task imposed by the context of any given working environment. We need to think clearly about the theory–practice relationship. What precisely does it mean to 'apply' theory to practice? Why would anyone want to do so? Under what circumstances is it actually desirable to do so? Without a clear answer to such questions a theorist simply has no business commenting on anybody's practices.

It is only by asking such questions that one can function as a philosopher. If my chapter has anything to offer practitioners, it is a note of caution in how they read the contributions of the other analysts, some of whom may be seasoned contributors to the debate about the prioritisation of health services. If I manage to say anything at all about this debate that is at once true and not positively harmful, then I will consider my modest goal for this chapter achieved.

Don't start here

There is a joke told about asking directions in certain parts of Ireland. Supposedly (though I have never experienced this myself) when you ask how to get to some well known landmark or vantage point, people will tell you 'well you don't start from here'. Far from being a silly answer, I find I can think of many circumstances when that is the best answer one could give. (But then I am part Irish.) Certainly, reading some of the descriptions of the cases I was asked to analyse for this chapter, my overwhelming reaction was that one does not start from here.

Consider the extremely valuable and in places extraordinarily moving account of a working day given by a practitioner who had to continuously reschedule appointments and make decisions about which visits to make personally and which responsibilities to delegate to voluntary workers she was helping to train and support. Of course, this person finishes work substantially later than planned, and despite feeling the children and families she worked with have received good care, she goes home feeling anxious about all the things that she has not had time to do (p. 29). Of course, the actual day looks nothing like the planned day (p. 26). She comments:

> I believe the most significant mistake I made on this day was not calling back the mothers who had left messages with office staff first thing in the morning. By relying on the team administrator to pass on their messages to me, I believe I wrongly prioritised the order of the visits. If I had spoken to the mother of the dying child personally, I might have been able to establish the urgency of the request for the visit. If I had decided to visit any later, this child might have died in pain (p. 28).

This is perhaps so, but in using her support staff in this way the practitioner was only following the advice with which health practitioners are constantly bombarded by such official sources of wisdom as the Clinical Governance Support Team, regarding being 'systems aware' and routinely relying on other members of one's team to communicate important messages. Such systematic reliance is explicitly advocated as excellent time management (Halligan *et al*. 2001). Yet when one traces this advice to its source, the contentious nature of the theorising behind it becomes apparent. Halligan and his associates reference three of the great 'gurus' of management theory: Crosby (1980), Deming (1986) and Juran (1964, 1974). Like so many official NHS publications, this is as crude an illustration of 'applying' theory to practice as one could hope to find: the application of theories of 'quality management' to the organisation of healthcare. Generalisations are derived from observations of how companies selling products like photocopiers increased their profits, and are then transferred to the context of healthcare, without even the acknowledgement that the change in context might have implications of a conceptual nature concerning what we mean by terms like 'quality' and 'excellence' (for examples, see Loughlin 2002a).

It is of course true that, in some cases, following this advice may indeed lead to excellent time management, but this case highlights the problems when one attempts to move from any apparently plausible generality to a highly specific situation. Here the practitioner concludes that she would have been better relying on her own experience and judgement to make a decision about what to do. Her reflection on these matters is valuable precisely because it is *her* reflection on *her own* experience. It does not follow that it is appropriate (intellectually or pragmatically) for someone commenting at a distance from her specific situation to offer her advice on how to handle such appalling demands on her time 'optimally'. She continues:

> However, while this is my own feeling, the family did not appear to share this. They expressed only gratitude that I had visited as they had requested (his mother had asked for a visit 'sometime today'). Written feedback from them since his death has confirmed that while the speed of the death had shocked them, they are positive about the peacefulness of his death and feel they were well supported in caring for their son at home, which was where he and they had desperately wanted to be. This feedback can surely be seen as a measure of success in relation to how prioritisation was managed in this instance (p. 28).

Certainly this reaction speaks well of the family, and undoubtedly reflects the excellent treatment they received from the practitioner, though the practitioner's inclination to characterise what this 'can be seen as' in the terms 'a measure of success in relation to how prioritisation was managed' perhaps indicates more about the current culture within the UK health service than it says about her relationship with the family. The language of prioritisation has permeated our thinking throughout the public sector. To have done our job well means, these days, to have 'prioritised' well. Yet as I read her account of the day I am struck by the obvious conclusion that there needs to be at least two of her to handle the workload she has. At the risk of repeating myself, she needs: more resources, more support, more time off, and I am quite sure that she both needs and certainly deserves better pay. To start one's thinking from the assumption that all of this is ruled out is simply to start in the wrong place, if one is to have anything to say that is at once true and worth saying.

What also struck me in the previous quotation is the family's (wholly admirable) failure to conform to a model of humanity derived from economic theory, and how that 'failure' meant that they only narrowly avoided the most terrible outcome of their child dying in pain. According to the crudest and least plausible versions of the economic model,[3] human beings are shamelessly self-interested operators, and if something is really important to them they will demand it, repeatedly and stridently. From this it follows logically that anyone not making such repeated and strident demands cannot have any urgent requirements to meet. The success of this model is quite extraordinary, and requires explanation because it is so patently false (Loughlin 2002a). Because of this model, when the doctor used to ask my elderly father how he was coping with his mobility problems and he said, truthfully, 'Well, I'm doing my best – I suppose I shouldn't complain', the doctor inferred that he had no serious problems, and as a result he and my mother suffered for years with inadequate support from the health service.

This family failed to 'talk up' the seriousness of their situation, probably because of an entirely human and reasonable disposition not to pester people or make too much of a fuss. We all know that for many people, asking for a visit 'sometime today' is about as demanding on an obviously over-stretched service as one can, in good conscience, bring oneself to be. One might be frightened to come across as 'bolshy', expecting one's claims to be met with some level of incredulity. As the practitioner says, on the basis of the family's communication with the administrator, she might well have decided to arrive later, and she was genuinely shocked to see how much worse the child was than she had anticipated (p. 27). Their failure to display the predictable behavioural traits of *homo economicus* nearly led to the most horrible outcome for this family because we are all, to some extent, in the grip of a false theory, which conditions us to make the wrong inferences at crucial times.

The same phenomenon comes across in the comments of parents whose children presented with perplexing and distressing problems.

I've been fighting for speech and language therapy for about twelve, thirteen years – parent of Katherine (p. 14), who eventually gained access to a therapist by lobbying her local Member of Parliament, after having initially been led to believe that there were 'just no therapists about'.

We had to fight for everything – parent of James (p. 20), who feels she was constantly 'fobbed off' and made to feel like she was exaggerating her child's problems.

What we have got for him we have had to push for which I found very frustrating – parent of Thomas (p. 24).

The stories of these parents indicate just how far the health economists and management theorists have won the battle for 'hearts and minds' (Donaldson 1999) in the health service against those service users who are perceived as typically overstating their needs. To reiterate: this perception is not based on evidence but rather it is generated by the theoretical assumptions of market economics – i.e. that most players in the social game are self-interested, and engaged in bidding for as big a piece of the pie as they can possibly get, so they cannot be trusted as sources of evidence when determining what they really need. Despite lacking an evidential basis, this assumption provides a rationale for downgrading the significance of what is frequently the best source of evidence available – patients reports of their own conditions and parents' reports of their children's conditions. So when we consider the alleged 'usefulness' of bringing economic theory to bear upon 'the problem' of how to distribute health resources, we need also to look critically at the extent to which this theoretical perspective helps to construct and contribute to the problem.

The other examples supplied are very much grist for the 'prioritising principles' mill. The discussion of paediatric physiotherapy services begins with a description of a series of events which may unfortunately sound all too familiar to many public sector workers. An increased workload for staff (p. 30) is followed not by an increase, but a decrease in the staffing base, resulting from the failure to replace a worker who leaves the school. The author notes that: 'The increasing caseload and the decrease in staffing meant that it was impossible to provide optimal levels of care to all children at the school' (p. 30).

The rest of the discussion concerns attempts to make the best of this (by implication) sub-optimal arrangement. In this respect (and despite some significant differences), it resembles the discussions of 'The least first framework' and 'Triage in speech and language therapy', the latter framing the debate most explicitly in terms derived from economic theory, speaking of demand outstripping supply and the subsequent need to manage resources efficiently and effectively (p. 35). It is worth noting that there is nothing *necessarily* wrong with this, since we always use some theoretical framework when discussing any issue. The important thing is to be aware of the framework and the way it shapes and conditions our thinking; to realise that its assumptions are by no means self-evident and may well be questioned and (as noted above) that some of the problems we are struggling with may be products of the very same framework that we are being encouraged to employ in their 'solution'. We must always keep open the possibility that a radical re-conceptualising of the problems might change the picture dramatically, recasting features of the situation as the real problem that had previously been treated as part of the background and, by implication, uncontentious.

To illustrate: if we approach the problem in each of the three examples in terms of 'how to prioritise' then we are making the following assumptions.

(a) The purpose of thinking about the problem isn't to explain it. The nature of the problem is self-explanatory, an empirical matter. Each discussion begins with a section called 'the background context', which describes the facts which led to *the problem* arising, so they seem to require no further comment or explanation.

(b) The really practical problem is the problem of how to make fair and rational prioritising decisions, given the background context. (This implies that if we can't say anything to help with that problem then we have nothing practical to say.)

Note that (a) and (b) serve to focus our attention on a part of the whole picture, diverting it away from the 'background context' which is therefore outside the scope of practical criticism. Again, this is not in itself a flaw in the approach, since all thinking requires that we select and isolate certain features of a situation and focus our attention upon them. But by treating the 'background context' as uncontroversial and insisting that we find a defensible solution to the 'practical problem', we assume that there is nothing about the background context that renders the problem unsusceptible to rational analysis and solution.

Why should that be so? It may well be that, given that background, no solution is more rational than any other, and whatever we do, someone will be the victim of an injustice: starting from here, we simply cannot be fair to all concerned. Consider: some slave societies are better and some are worse than others, but they are all unjust. So if our starting point is a slave society and that 'background context' is outside the scope of our discussion, we simply cannot arrive at a solution to the problem of how to organise the production of life's necessities that is 'fair to all concerned'. Why should we just assume that our own place in history is so much more fortunate, that given this starting point we can find rational and fair solutions to our social problems without fundamental social change? Is it not even possible that our current social and economic arrangements – with all of the inequality and suffering they necessitate – are the real problem, in the same way that (most of us readily accept) the underlying social and economic arrange- ments in many earlier human societies were the true obstacles to justice and social progress?[4]

Such possibilities would be taken seriously by (amongst others) theorists adopting a Marxist approach. Marx would focus on the background, looking beyond the 'background contexts' the authors describe to the broader economic environment – regarding it as needing explaining and indeed as being the real problem. Given the background of a monstrously unfair economic system that disproportionately benefits some and leaves much of the world dispossessed,[5] it is absurd to hope to take some sector of the economy (say the health service) in isolation from the rest of the world and render it 'fair and rational'. One must of course try to be as fair as possible in one's dealings with others (surely another banality!) but the real problems for the provision of health services, and indeed for the way we provide for all of our most basic needs, extend so far beyond our particular work contexts that it is hardly surprising that working life often feels like a constant struggle against overwhelming irrational forces: that is what it is! (Loughlin 2002a)

On this approach, the cases described in Chapters 2–4 serve to demonstrate the true effects of broader economic factors on public sector workers and service users. Since labour produces excess value, an increasing workload will be a pattern that emerges as resources shrink to allow profits to be maintained. So the worker who officially finishes at 5 pm in fact finishes at 6.15 (p. 26) and this 'cost' (the portion of her life consistently stolen from her) remains uncounted, invisible and therefore uncompensated. The physiotherapists take on functions previously performed by an occupational therapist (p. 30 *re.* physiotherapy services example) and in general it becomes the responsibility of practitioners to solve problems that are obviously not of their making. Workers will do their best to create solutions appropriate to the contexts of their work, but it is not the job of theory to construct broad rationalisations for the arrangements that create the problems. And whether they intend it or not, that is what most academic contributors to the prioritising debate – be they economists, organisational theorists or indeed moral philosophers – actually do, since what they set out to prove is that, given this economic starting point, a fair and rational organisation of society is indeed possible:

> While the Western powers can find any amount of money to fund bombardments of countries whose leaders have fallen out of favour, as far as health resources are concerned economic scarcity is a 'fact of life', so governments search for rationales to deny access to those services to some groups within the population. It is currently unfashionable to give a Marxist analysis of any social phenomenon. Even so, it is perhaps worth pointing out that what is in origin an *economic* problem for governments has (as a Marxist might expect) given rise to a flurry of intellectual activity in the field of *moral philosophy*, as academics construct theories of justice in resource allocation to prove that fair methods do in fact exist to ration essential health resources as (it just so happens) the economy requires.
>
> (Loughlin 2002a)

The Boss's Helper and the Self-Help Therapist are both theorists who tell workers to stop moaning about the fact that they lack sufficient resources to do their jobs properly, and to focus on how to prioritise given the world as it is. They rationalise this by observing that it is 'unreasonable' to keep asking for better resources, more support, more money and more time off, since if everyone insisted on being properly resourced then the system would collapse: 'we' 'cannot afford' even to provide proper support to workers whose job is to prevent children from dying in great pain. But if that is so, then it only serves to prove the Marxist point that the economic system, the 'world as it is', is the cause of the problem: we need a new world.

As I have argued this point in the text already cited I will not recap the arguments in detail here. My point for the moment is simply to note that, if one rejects the assumptions of classic economics in favour of an alternative approach, such as Marxism, then the discussion of 'prioritising'[6] is not pointless. The cases discussed are still eminently worthy of attention, but the point of discussing them changes. The point then is to focus on the unfairness and irrationality of the rules of the game – to call for a new game, not to tell anyone how to win the game as it stands because it is unwinnable. The best one can hope for is survival and the project of changing the game is not one that can be achieved in a working day, nor even in a lifetime: it is one of the many things we cannot do alone because it takes generations.

All one can do 'as a philosopher' is encourage the practice of constantly questioning one's underlying assumptions, and noting the practical import of them in specific situations. (See, for instance, the impact of market economic assumptions on how we interpret people's expressions of need, noted above.) There are more profound and underlying questions about how we can possibly determine which theoretical assumptions are true, or best, in any given context. I am by no means inclined to avoid those questions, or understate their importance, or dismiss them as mere matters of opinion, and indeed I discuss them in more depth elsewhere (Loughlin 2002a, 2004b). But in the space available here it will have to be enough to note that, if one wants to think about how to practice, then there is no clear line at which that thinking process comes to a halt. Certainly anyone reading a book like this in the hope of finding a checklist of principles to follow to produce better practices is not only likely to be disappointed: they should realise that their disappointment is based on the fact that, perhaps influenced by some of the questionable theories that shape the prioritising debate, they have started their thinking in the wrong place.

Notes

1 This is an extremely conservative estimate, likely to be accepted (albeit reluctantly) by even the most determined apologists for the 'free market'. It of course depends on how one interprets 'preventable' and 'poverty', but more realistic estimates place the figure at nearer to 30,000 child deaths *per day* from wholly preventable, poverty-related disease and malnutrition (UNICEF 2000).

2 I am not, of course, suggesting that academic jargon renders advice insightful – rather, cloaked in impressive-sounding jargon, very mundane 'insights' can appear more profound than they are.

3 The ones that, along with a lot of quack 'motivational' psychology, have had the most influence on the contemporary 'management science' already referred to, that has shaped the nature of life in the public sector for so long now.

4 In popular debate, we apply this point not only to societies at earlier points in history than our own, but increasingly to societies in the present deemed less advanced than ours. Our current leaders are particularly fond of claiming that social progress cannot happen in other parts of the world until countries embrace a UK/US model of 'democracy' as a basis for all social arrangements, as well as economic arrangements which (coincidentally, we are assured) are highly compatible with Western business interests.

5 To test the intuition that the current economic system is a just one, try to think that it is while re-reading footnote 1.

6 Or, as it used to be called, 'rationing' – and please note that this terminological shift also has ideological underpinnings (Loughlin 2002a).

References

Beauchamp, T.L. and Childress, J.F. (2001) *Principles of Biomedical Ethics*. New York: Oxford University Press.

Crosby, P.B. (1980) *Quality is Free*. New York: Penguin.

Deming, W.E. (1986) *Out of the Crisis*. Cambridge: Cambridge University Press.

Donaldson, L. (1999) 'Clinical governance – medical practice in a new era', *The Journal of The Medical Defense Union*, **15**, 7–9.

Halligan, A., Nicholls, S. and O'Neill, S. (2001) 'Clinical Governance: developing organisational capability', in A. Miles, P. Hill and B. Hurwitz (eds.) *Clinical Governance and the NHS Reforms*. London: Aesculapius Medical Press.

Juran, J.M. (1964) *Managerial Breakthrough*. New York: McGraw-Hill.

Juran, J.M. (1974) *Quality Control Handbook*. New York: McGraw-Hill.

Kottow, M.H. (2004) 'Whither bioethics? A reply to commentaries on "The rationale of value-laden medicine"', *Journal of Evaluation in Clinical Practice*, **10**: 71–3.

Loughlin, M. (2002a) *Ethics, Management and Mythology: Rational Decision Making for Health Service Professionals*. Oxford: Radcliffe Medical Press.

Loughlin, M. (2002b) 'Arguments at cross-purposes: moral epistemology and medical ethics', *Journal of Medical Ethics*, **28**: 28–32.

Loughlin, M. (2004a) 'Orwellian quality – the bosses' revolution', in M. Learmonth and N. Harding (eds.) *Unmasking Health Management – a Critical Text*. New York: Nova Science/Hauppauge.

Loughlin, M. (2004b) 'Management, science and reality', *Philosophy of Management*, **4**: 35–44.

Loughlin, M. (2004c) 'Camouflage is still no defence – another plea for a straight answer to the question "what is bioethics?"', *Journal of Evaluation in Clinical Practice*, **10**: 75–83.

Moss, M. (2003) 'Practically useless? Why management theory needs Popper', *Philosophy of Management*, **3**: 31–42.

Seedhouse, D.F. (1996) 'Philosophy must fall to Earth', *Health Care Analysis*, **4**: 91–4.

UNICEF (2000) 'Progress of Nations 2000', New York: UNICEF.

Chapter 10

Professional judgement and decision making

Margaret Miers

Introduction

Prioritisation involves individuals making judgements and decisions. The aims of the study of professional judgement and decision making are to understand how professionals make judgements and decisions and how they could, or perhaps should, make better decisions. The emphasis is often not so much on the outcomes of a decision but on the processes of judgement and decision making. Such an interest, although only relatively recently identified as a distinct subject area of interdisciplinary study (the Society for Judgement and Decision Making was founded in 1986), has long fascinated philosophers, psychologists, management and political scientists as well as lawyers, policy makers and health professionals. This chapter first outlines different approaches to studying professional judgement and decision making and then reviews the case studies in the light of the approaches introduced.

Connolly, Arkes and Hammond (2000) identify two main reasons for the emergence of the study of judgement and decision making in the 1960s. First, amongst psychologists, the credibility of both stimulus–response behaviourism and Freudian psychology declined, giving way to a shift in research interest towards 'mental activity'. Second, the arrival of computers enabled modelling of mental activity and the development of research into 'human information processing' and artificial intelligence. Connolly and associates describe two different approaches to representing judgement and decision making, one 'looking forward' and the other 'looking backward':

> *decision analysis* – which involves an *a priori* decomposition of the decision process – and, second, . . . *judgement analysis* – which involves an *a posteriori* decomposition of the judgement process. (p. 3)

The distinction between decision analysis and judgement analysis is, as the authors acknowledge, somewhat arbitrary. Both approaches accept that professional judgement and decision making are processes characterised by uncertainty. O'Sullivan (1999), writing about social work, illuminates this point, describing decisions as problematic balancing acts, based on incomplete information, within time constraints, under pressure from different sources, with uncertainty as to the likely outcome of the different options, and the constant fear that something will go wrong. (p.3)

Judgement can be seen as the process by which necessary inputs for decisions in relation to options, uncertainties and values are made. Judgement analysis, therefore, complements decision analysis.

Decision analysis

Decision analysis involves decomposing a decision process into components. It is applied in situations where alternative actions (options) are available and there is uncertainty about possible outcomes and the 'best' course of action (depending on judgements made about the desirability of the different possible outcomes). The components are: (i) options/alternatives; (ii) outcomes; (iii) likelihoods or probabilities and (iv) utilities. Decision analysis provides a procedure for synthesising the components through a diagram, which structures the decision process.

Decision Trees

The value of a decision tree is in clarifying the components and presenting a way of identifying the optimal choice, assumed to be that which gives the best chance of a good outcome, or, in the language of decision analysis, maximises expected utility. To construct a decision tree, the decision maker needs information about each of the four components:

1. What are all the possible courses of action/inaction i.e. what are the options?
2. What are the possible events (outcomes) that might follow from courses of actions or inaction?
3. What is the probability of each final outcome?
4. What is the value (utility/disutility) of each final outcome?

None of the questions above is easy to answer, particularly specifying probabilities and the value of the outcomes. However, the structure of a decision tree may help to clarify the components of decisions such as those set out in Hayhow's least first framework (Chapter 8). Hayhow discusses the difficulties of decisions around early stuttering, arising from the high rate of natural recovery and because of the dangers of treatment raising anxiety and exacerbating the difficulty with fluency. Treatment will involve some costs as well as benefits. The health professional may be best placed to assess the likelihood of treatment leading to improvements; however, it is the individual who stutters (and other interested parties such as relatives and carers) whose utilities matter. Figure 10.1 illustrates the possible treatment options and outcomes. It hypothesises the likelihood that each outcome will occur and the value of each outcome on a scale of 1–100. Practitioners can use their clinical experience and data from the literature to propose these probabilities. Asking the client seems to be the easiest way of assigning a value or a utility to each outcome.

Figure 10.1 shows how the *expected utility* of each outcome is calculated by multiplying its probability of occurring by its utility. The *expected utility* of each option is the sum of the expected utilities of each outcome on the option's 'branches' of the decision tree. In this instance, 'treat' is the option that will maximise expected utility. It should be remembered that this example is provided purely to illustrate a decision tree and that a real analysis of the decision in detail would produce more reasonable hypotheses about the probabilities and utilities.

Probability judgements

Heuristics and biases

One area of judgement and decision-making research, 'behavioural decision theory', has explored the notion of 'bounded or limited rationality' (Dowie and Elstein 1988). The assumption is that our capacity for rational thought is limited by our capacity to remember and process information. Hence we find ways ('heuristics') to reduce the mental strain involved. A considerable body of research has explored common errors in judgement under uncertainty. Tversky and Kahneman (1974) explored common 'rules of thumb' or 'heuristics' that lead to errors in estimating probabilities and identified three key sources of error. Availability bias refers to the fact that we often assess the probability of an event by the ease with which instances of its occurrence come to mind. Availability bias explains why we can be significantly influenced by what is in the news. Anchoring bias occurs when we fail to move beyond our first thought, sticking to our initial formulation of the problem and failing to reassess assumptions in the light of new information. Representativeness bias can lead to serious errors, particularly through ignoring base rates. In answering a common probabilistic question, 'what is the probability that object A belongs to class B?' people rely on the extent to which A resembles B. For example, if A is a shy individual wearing glasses and we are asked to assess the probability that A's occupation is one of the following: farmer, airline pilot, shop assistant, librarian, we are likely to choose 'librarian' since characteristics of A are seen as similar to the stereotype of that occupation. The error we have made is ignoring the significance of the base rate frequency. There are many more shop assistants in the population than there are librarians. There has been considerable debate, however, about the nature and significance of these identified 'errors', as well as about the details of the underpinning research studies (Edwards and von Winterfeldt 2000; Gigerenzer and Goldstein 1996).

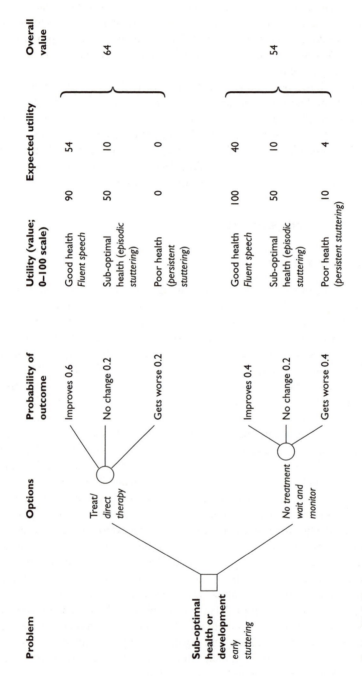

Figure 10.1 Decision tree

One widely observed and accepted bias, however, is hindsight bias, in which we exaggerate what could have been anticipated in foresight (Fischhoff 1975). This can easily be corrected by writing down our judgements before an event occurs or before we learn the answer. The doctor involved in the case of Thomas demonstrates hindsight bias when she learns that Thomas has developmental co-ordination disorder. Thomas's mother records the doctor's response as 'Oh yes, its developmental co-ordination disorder, oh yes I can understand that' and comments 'well if she could understand that why couldn't you have seen it when we first brought him?' (p. 24)

The Bayesian approach and Bayes' theorem

The advantage of decision analysis lies in its combination of a structured approach to clarifying thinking and its use of numbers and calculation to make visible the weightings used in arriving at a choice (Miers 1990). Understanding human 'bounded rationality' can help individuals understand their own thinking. Decision analysts argue that individuals can be helped to maximise expected utility by elicitation and computation such as Bayes' theorem. From the Bayesian perspective, probabilities of events occurring are not 'out there', capable of estimation using 'objective' methods. Probabilities are subjective. Individuals assess probabilities on the basis of their own knowledge and beliefs and an individual's assessment of a probability *for* (rather than *of*) an event occurring is an expression of a view rather than a 'scientific' appraisal of social processes or properties of the physical world. Bayes' theorem states that a posterior opinion that a hypothesis is true is the product of a prior opinion multiplied by the likelihood ratio of the obtained data/information given that the hypothesis is true. It is a far more accurate way of calculating probabilities on the basis of additional information than relying on our mental short cuts.

Judgement analysis

Judgement analysis has similar advantages to decision analysis. Judgement analysis, however, concentrates on identifying the components of a decision after a series of judgements have been made. Judgement is seen as a cognitive process in which a person draws an inference about something that cannot be seen. Inferences are made from cues. The case studies in Part II provide a range of examples of uncertainties over the meaning of cues. Mothers report screaming, pulling legs up in pain, projectile vomiting, differences in appearance (ear, temples), failure to make any sounds, limited growth; all cues that add to concern about a child. Professionals assess through a variety of tests (kidney scans, EEG, CAT scan, hearing and vision tests). Inferences drawn from the cues differ. Mothers perceive 'something wrong' whilst professionals are seen as minimising the significance of cues as, for example, 'only colic' (Katherine, p. 14) and sometimes maximising the likelihood of negative outcomes, predicting a child will 'never walk, never talk'

(Katherine, p. 14). Central to judgement analysis is a recognition of the 'problem' of inaccuracies in any cue interpretation or any test result. Subsequent (gold standard) information often reveals that positive or negative test results are misleading. Further testing (or the passage of time), for example, reveals that a child described as a slow reader does not have dyslexia, as may have been hypothesised, or that a child does have a disorder, as may have been denied.

Any threshold value on any test used to aid judgement will yield false positives and false negatives. Knowing the sensitivity (the true positive rate) and specificity (true negative rate) of a test is therefore important. The case study on James illustrates the difficulties in determining threshold values of a cue or range of cues for the presence or absence of a condition. There were considerable difficulties and contradictory judgements around diagnosing FG syndrome.

In medical decision making doctors arrive at diagnoses by considering the results of a range of diagnostic tests, their own physical examinations and the information they gain from patients. They will assign more weight to some of these cues than others (with more or less understanding of the predictive value of test results i.e. the likelihood of a condition being present if the test is positive or not being present if the test is negative). It is interesting to note that Katherine, James and Thomas all have their eyesight monitored more closely by professionals than parents thought necessary. Doctors are trained to monitor and place weight on biophysical signs.

Judgement analysis seeks to understand how cue data are organised into a judgement. Although individual decision makers may think they use information in a complex manner, one research theme suggested that humans process information in a straightforward way, represented by a linear model, in which judgements are formulated as a simple weighted sum of the values of the cues used. A common finding has been that judgements are made on the basis of a relatively small number of cues. Furthermore, this area of research has found that there are often significant differences between the weights individuals say they are giving to information (cues) and the weights they appear to be using when cues and decisions are 'captured' and analysed statistically (Kirwan et al. 1983; Fisch et al. 1981). Judgement research has led to the development of data-based aids based on judgement analyses. These aids draw on statistical reasoning such as regression equations or Bayes' theorem. One example of an early decision aid used in clinical practice was a database compiled to support clinical judgements about abdominal pain (de Dombal 1974; Adams et al. 1986). The database could calculate the likelihood ratios for a set of signs and symptoms related to abdominal pain and generate a probability of someone presenting with a set of signs and symptoms having a particular condition such as appendicitis. Sadly the system was judged to be 'unacceptable' by clinicians and has never been integrated into clinical practice.

Understanding expertise

Findings from research have cast considerable doubt on the efficacy of human judgement when making decisions without paying attention to systematic analysis. Nevertheless, despite evidence of flaws in human cognition, professionals still usually make judgements and decisions by processing information in their heads, and prefer to do so. One argument for this approach is the view that expertise resides in the ability to synthesise information and experience without recourse to formal analysis. Accordingly, some analysts have concentrated on attempting to model the judgement process of experts by reproducing and studying problem-solving behaviour, often using computers. Others have focused on 'process tracing' using verbal report methodologies in an attempt to extract the expertise. The use of the resulting algorithms and protocols as aids to judgement and decision making is becoming widespread in clinical practice. Hayhow describes the least first framework as an aid to decision making about stuttering.

Unfortunately it may be impossible to extract and model the key elements of expertise. Schön (1983) has argued that, although professions are deemed to have a systematic knowledge base, the application of that knowledge base in the context of everyday professional judgements and decisions is based on 'knowing-in-action'. Some professions have areas of practice in which practitioners can function as technical experts, drawing upon systematically collected evidence to inform practice. Other professions, with less well established knowledge bases, practise in areas where there is not a systematic body of evidence to inform their judgements. Practitioners work in 'the swampy lowlands' (Schön 1983), dealing with 'messy but crucially important problems and, when asked to describe their methods of inquiry, they speak of experience, trial and error, intuition and muddling through' (p.43).

Schön's work draws attention to the importance of a professional's tacit knowing-in-action. Professionals display skills in their everyday practice that they cannot necessarily explain. On a daily basis they face new and troubling experiences, which they try to make sense of, and through that sense-making process, they reflect on the understandings implicit in action and thus surface these understandings, which are reviewed, restructured and embodied in further action. Schön sees this 'reflection-in-action' as central to the 'art' of professional practice. Schön's work has supported and generated an enormous literature on 'reflective practice' and widespread acceptance of the importance of the 'reflective practitioner'. One of the advantages of 'knowledge-in-action' is that it leads to rapid judgement and decision making and thus can seem an efficient use of professional expertise. Critics would argue that such individualised judgements lead to sub-optimal treatment, inequities and error.

Dreyfus and Dreyfus (1986) have supported the significance of experts and expertise. They have suggested that the stages of developing expertise involve progressively less dependence on analytical approaches to identifying elements of a situation, less attention to acting on the elements and less reliance on others for help in recognising the significance of the whole situation. Experts' ability to appreciate the whole situation supports an ability to make decisions and to plan in order to attain goals. Katherine's mother sees her daughter's paediatrician as an expert to be trusted partly because of her ability to see the whole picture. She 'knows her stuff', Katherine 'has been seeing her for many years' and she 'co-ordinates it all' (Katherine p. 16). The Dreyfuses see the novice as reliant on analysis; expertise is gradually acquired step by step, through analysis of components. Experts discard analysis. Their thinking is intuitive. In nursing, Benner (1984) drew upon the work of Dreyfus and Dreyfus in her own analysis of acquisition of expertise through the Dreyfuses' stages of skill acquisition: novice; advanced beginner; competent; proficient; expert. The children's palliative care specialist nurse regretted that she had not called back the mothers who had left messages because she felt that if she had spoken to the mother of the dying child personally she 'might have been able to establish the urgency of the request for the visit' (p. 28). She had confidence that her experience and expertise would have made a difference. Benner's work led to a prolonged emphasis in the nursing literature on description, exploration and celebration of nursing 'know-how' or intuition acquired through experience, and to widespread adoption of the stages of skill acquisition in education programmes. Benner claimed:

> the expert nurse perceives the situation as a whole, uses past concrete situations as paradigms, and moves to the accurate region of the problem without wasteful consideration of a large number of irrelevant options.
>
> (Benner 1984, p.3)

If such a process seems effortless in execution, that is perceived, as in creative arts, as sign of supreme skill. Debates about the relative merits of analysis and intuition have been supplemented by a growing literature on professional education. Such literature has explored the development, use and significance of 'tacit' knowledge. Tacit knowledge builds with experience and differs from explicit knowledge (Eraut 2000). Tacit knowledge comes through learning 'on the job' and may become more explicit through a process of reflection. The case studies in Part II illustrate both professionals and parents reflecting on, and surfacing, their tacit knowledge. Mothers talk about 'knowing something was not quite right'.

The cognitive continuum framework

Hammond (1978, 1980, 1981, Hamm 1988) avoids an 'intuition versus analysis' approach through viewing analysis and intuition not as opposing forms of judgement but as modes of cognition at different ends of a cognitive continuum. The cognitive continuum 'framing' enables us to see that most of our cognitive activity involves elements of both analysis and intuition. Hammond described six modes of cognition, which are used at different times depending on the extent to which a judgement/decision 'task' is ill-structured or well-structured, the time available to consider the task and the possibility of processing different components of the task in different ways, e.g. through discussion with peers or use of a protocol, an algorithm or a computerised data analysis package. Hammond's six modes of cognition are: scientific experiment; controlled trial; quasi experiment; system-aided judgement; peer-aided judgement and intuitive judgement.

Dowie (2003) has extended the continuum to include a seventh mode of cognition that does not involve cognitive judgement and is based on emotion (see Figure 10.2). His advocacy of the cognitive continuum framework emphasises that a key difference between analysis and intuition is explicitness. Making components of judgements and decisions explicit opens them up to discussion and provides opportunities for peer review and debate. It can also reveal variation in practice amongst peers. Roulstone (2001) explored consensus and variation amongst speech and language therapists in the initial assessment of preschool children. She found consensus around relative priority of children, categories informing assessment and interpretations of incoming information. There were variations in preferred methods of assessment, thresholds of concern and interventions offered. Roulstone argues that 'differences should be acknowledged, carefully documented and their reasons made explicit as far as possible' (p. 347). Dowie has extensively argued the case for greater use of decision analysis to support clarity and openness in professional judgement.

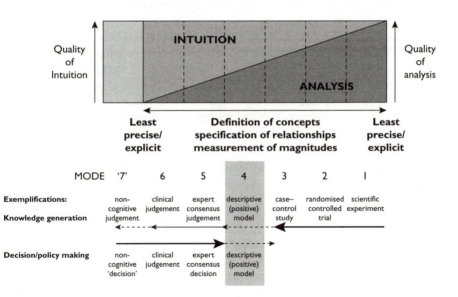

Figure 10.2 The cognitive continuum framework

Source: In Dowie, J. (2003) Health impact: its estimation assessment and analysis. Chapter 18 in Orme, J. *et al. Public Health for the 21st Century: New perspectives on policy, participation and practice,* Open University Press, Maidenhead p. 303. (Reproduced with kind permission of the Open University Press.)

Reflections on case studies

Three main issues raised by the case studies are noteworthy in the context of discussing professional judgement and decision making. First is the perennial difficulty of dealing with information/cues/data. Second is the nature and significance of 'expertise' and third the significance of explicitness in decisions, relationships and prioritisation.

Dealing with complex and uncertain information

The case studies present many examples of uncertainty around the significance of information. Negative aspects of such uncertainty include the fact that mothers suffered from a perception that their own behaviour could be seen as part of a set of diagnostic cues. Vigilance and concern about a child's health could be seen as a sign of mental illness in a mother. Parents were frustrated by a lack of communication about the process of judgement and decision making, that is the process of using information to decide on priorities and actions. Professional knowledge can lead to an emphasis on the relevance of physical cues rather than more social cues reported by the parents. Professional assessment of probabilities about potential often appeared particularly pessimistic, although such pessimism may be motivated by the unspoken need to prioritise. Probability assessments are not communicated or shared, suggesting that they are made intuitively and implicitly, if at all.

In contrast, some professionals provide specialist services that pay attention to individual needs, are responsive to new information, including information from families, and are able to adapt services, for example by changing the time of an optician appointment to lower the likelihood of distress (Katherine p. 6). The children's palliative care nurse shows her own adaptability on a day when needs led her to reprioritise activities and reorganise a planned day (Chapter 5). The mother of Katherine praises both the optician and a speech and language therapy assistant for a responsive approach to information and complexity.

The complexity of James's needs increases the probability of complications associated with any treatment. Professionals anticipating potential difficulties severely delays treatment for toothache. Whereas in specialist palliative care services children with the most complex needs appear to receive priority, in other areas complexity leads to service difficulties and delays. The description of the triage system in speech and language therapy (Chapter 7), however, suggests that a structured approach to prioritisation and decision making allowed a service to face difficulties with waiting lists, complaints and inequities successfully. The complexities were analysed and explicit guidelines drawn up. The professional case studies suggest that adoption of formal modelling (stage 4 on the cognitive continuum) assists the handling of information, uncertainty and prioritisation.

Expertise

However, the case studies also demonstrate that professionals and parents place a high value on expertise. The specialist nurse's regret at relying on an administrator's report of a telephone conversation rather than making her own assessment has already been mentioned. Clearly the nurse had confidence in her own communicative ability and saw expert communication skills as important in assessment and judgement. It is interesting to note that experienced professionals are used to triaging speech and language therapy referrals. Experienced therapists meet parents, listen to their concerns and gather initial information. They observe parent and child using a two-way mirror, 'providing a rapid insight into expressive language and play' (p. 37). Decisions are reached with the parent and child. The success of the triage system seems to support the argument that experience brings a level of expertise that allows professionals to understand the whole picture more quickly than a novice. Communicative ability may be at the heart of such expertise. Nevertheless, prioritising in triage is underpinned by clarity about key relevant factors, bringing structured analysis into the decision-making process.

Explicitness

The triage case study (Chapter 7) illustrates the importance of explicitness as well as expertise. Parents are asked for their views about referral and urgency, presumably necessitating a discussion of relevant cues and possible outcomes. Croot (Chapter 6) reports that physiotherapists found that once the judgements were made more explicit, they could make the reasons for treatment priorities explicit to others and they were more confident in explaining their professional judgement. Assessment and goal setting was regularly discussed with others (e.g. parents and school staff) as well as physiotherapy colleagues. This allowed physiotherapists to negotiate timings of treatment with the wider team.

In contrast, the case study of Katherine suggests that many professionals involved did not appear to discuss the support provided for Katherine. Katherine's mother is clear that she would like professionals to be more explicit.

> 'I would like to have a report of the findings of the assessment and give an input. And have an opportunity to discuss it. And then when the programme goes into place then to be able to see the programme, see what's happening, what's working and have a say really. Then when further assessment is done see what progress has been made' (p. 15).

The mothers in all the case studies are clear that they would like professionals to communicate more, more effectively and more explicitly. One area in which professionals appear to continue to largely rely on unspoken and subjective assumptions is values. The case studies show many examples of a lack of awareness on the part of the professionals of the value placed on activities and information by the families involved. Most striking is, in the case study of Katherine, the lack of awareness on the part of the professionals and service providers about the value the family placed on treatment. Families' lack of information about the availability and variability of services suggests limited attempts on the part of service providers to explain the competing pressures on professional time and resources. There is a lack of a shared dialogue about priorities. Understandably, parents prioritise their own child and perceive themselves as battling with professionals who think they are on the same side. The dilemmas are encapsulated by Katherine's mother's feelings:

> 'I feel that Katherine is my priority. If I don't fight for her rights then there's no-one else who will do it for me, I just want her to have the best. So that she can develop to the best of her potential. If that means fighting for a service she's rightfully entitled to then that's the way it's going to be . . . I am willing to do that for her' (p. 16).

Conclusion

Overall the case studies suggest that there is some movement towards greater analysis and away from individual intuition in professional judgement, as is advocated in the literature on decision making. Analysis makes professionals more explicit about their judgements, and supports increased communication between members of teams and parents, children and carers. The case studies suggest that this is what families are asking for, and presumably the children themselves, although there is little information in the case studies about the views of children and young people. Nevertheless, expertise remains valued. Is the 'explicit expert' the professional of the future?

There are no clear answers to questions such as 'what is best for Katherine?' or 'What are her entitlements?' but the study of professional judgement and decision making can offer alternative ways of thinking and practical tools to help constructive and open debate. Identifying our probability assessments and clarifying the values we place on different outcomes would be a major move forward. Decision analysis asks us to look deeply and explicitly at what might be 'the best' and for whom. Familiarity with the literature on professional judgement and decision making would support and challenge professional practice in the twenty-first century.

References

Adams, I.D., Chan, M., Clifford, P.C., Cooke, W. M., Dallos, V., de Dombal, F.T., Edwards, M.H., Hancock, D.M., Hewett, D.J., McIntyre, N., Somerville, P.G., Spiegelhalter, D.J., Wellwood, J. and Wilson, D.H. (1986) 'Computer aided diagnosis of acute abdominal pain: a multicentre study', *British Medical Journal*, **293**: 800–4.

Benner, P. (1984) *From Novice to Expert: Excellence and Power in Clinical Nursing Practice*. Menlo Park, California: Addison Wesley.

Connolly, T., Arkes, H.R. and Hammond, K.R. (eds) (2000) *Judgement and Decision Making* (2nd edn). Cambridge: Cambridge University Press.

de Dombal, F.T., Leaper, D.J., Horrocks, J.C., Staniland, J.R. and McCann, A.P. (1974) 'Human and computer-aided diagnosis of abdominal pain: Further report with emphasis on performance of clinicians', *British Medical Journal* 1: 376–80.

Dowie, J. (2003) Health impact: its estimation assessment and analysis. Chapter 18 in Orme, J., Powell, J., Taylor, P., Harrison, T. and Grey, M., *Public Health for the 21st Century: New perspectives on policy, participation and practice*. Maidenhead: Open University Press, pp. 296–309.

Dowie, J. and Elstein, A. (eds) (1988) *Professional Judgement: A reader in clinical decision making*. Cambridge: Cambridge University Press.

Dreyfus, H.L. and Dreyfus, S.E. (1986) *Mind over Machine: The Power of Human Intuition and Expertise in the era of the Computer*. New York: The Free Press.

Edwards, W. and von Winterfeldt, D. (2000) On Cognitive Illusions and the Implications. In Connolly, T., Arkes, H.R. and Hammond, K.R. (eds) *Judgement and Decision Making* (2nd edn). Cambridge: Cambridge University Press, pp. 592–620.

Eraut, M. (2000) 'Non-formal learning and tacit knowledge in professional work', *British Journal of Educational Psychology* 70: 113–36.

Fisch, H.-U., Hammond, K.R., Joyce, C.R.B. and O'Reilly, M. (1981) 'An experimental study of the clinical judgement of general physicians in evaluating and prescribing for depression', *British Journal of Psychiatry* 138: 100–9.

Fischhoff, B. (1975) 'Hindsight ≠ Foresight: the effect of outcome knowledge on judgement under uncertainty', *Journal of Experimental Psychology: Human Perception and Performance*, I, 288–99.

Gigerenzer, G. and Goldstein, D.G. (1996) 'Reasoning the fast and frugal way: Models of Bounded Rationality', *Psychological Review*, 103: 650–70.

Hamm, R.M. (1988) Clinical Intuition and Clinical Analysis: Expertise and the Cognitive Continuum. In Dowie, J. and Elstein, A. (eds) (1988) *Professional Judgement: A reader in clinical decision making*. Cambridge: Cambridge University Press, pp. 78–105.

Hammond, K.R. (1978) Toward increasing competence of thought in public policy formation. In Hammond, K.R. (ed.) *Judgement and Decision in Public Policy Formation*. Boulder, Colorado: Westview Press, pp. 11–32.

Hammond, K.R. (1980) *The integration of research in judgement and decision theory* (Report # 226). Boulder, University of Colorado, Centre for Research on Judgement and Policy.

Hammond, K.R. (1981) *Principles of organisation in intuitive and analytical cognition*. (Report # 231). Boulder, University of Colorado, Centre for Research on Judgement and Policy.

Kirwan, J.R., Chaput de Santoigne, D.M., Joyce, C.R.B. and Currey, H.L.F. (1983) 'Clinical judgement in rheumatoid arthritis. II Judging "current disease activity" in clinical practice', *Annals of the Rheumatic Diseases*, 42: 648–651.

Miers, M. (1990) 'Developing skills in decision making', *Nursing Times* 86(30): 32–3.

O'Sullivan, T. (1999) *Decision Making in Social Work*. Basingstoke: Palgrave.

Roulstone, S. (2001) 'Consensus and variation between speech and language therapists in the assessment and selection of preschool children for intervention: a body of knowledge or idiosyncratic decisions?' *International Journal of Language and Communication Disorders*. **36(3)**: 329–48.

Schön, D. (1983) *The Reflective Practitioner: How Professionals Think in Action*. New York: Basic Books.

Tversky, A. and Kahneman, D. (1974) 'Judgement Under Uncertainty: Heuristics and Biases', *Science* **185**: 1124–31.

Chapter 11

The view from the 'dismal science'

Paul Rowlands

Epidemic, pestilence and plague with inevitable famine stalking in the rear was the future for mankind predicted by economist Thomas Malthus in 1798:[1] resources to feed mankind would grow slower than the number of mouths to feed. The result, no matter how good man became at setting priorities, was the dismal vision set out above. However, not for the last time, history proved an economist's predictions wrong.

Economists have continued to try to predict human behaviour, despite these early setbacks. These attempted predictions are used to rearrange our available resources to get the best out of what we have at the time. Nowadays these predictions are usually, but not always, more accurate than poor old Malthus's. Economists have two approaches to studying human behaviour. The first looks at the individual (or groups of individuals) and how they behave when making a decision, how they behave when faced with a choice. The second approach looks at organisations (such as governments or NHS trusts) and how they allocate resources amongst competing demands on a grander, more global scale.

Whether we look at behaviour on the grand, global scale or from the perspective of the individual, we face the same problem. We can't have everything. It matters not if you are a born-again Puritan or a rabid, consumer hedonist, there will be things (or services) you would like to have, but cannot, because your resources don't stretch that far. The same is true for the richest global organisations bestriding the world and bullying poor, benighted politicians everywhere. They also have to make decisions between what to have and what not to have, or at least, what to have now and what to postpone until some time in the future.

Thus the core of an 'economic' approach to an issue is the study of how people set about prioritising the choices they have to make.[2] A generalisation from the two centuries or so of economics is that these priorities can be set in two broad ways. Priorities can be set by each individual or group that forms the 'market' for the service – a market approach (the classic market system). Alternatively, the priorities can be set by someone who is only indirectly involved (e.g. the government or a planning group) directing what 'should' be done. This is a command approach. Extreme examples of this command approach would be the USSR, Hitler's Third Reich or even Churchill's UK war economy in the early and mid-1940s. In fact,

Aneurin Bevan founded the NHS in 1948 as a centralised, unitary 'command' system. This idea didn't survive first contact with the medical profession. Clearly nowadays the NHS (and most of the world) is a mixture of both approaches. Some markets are more 'directed' than others even in the same country. Also some countries have a tendency to direct more parts of their economy than others (e.g. Cuba under Castro). The actual proportions of command and market systems in each 'mixed economy' vary. The proportions also change over time. The UK became less command- and more market-lead during the 1980s and 1990s. There is no one 'third way', a phrase beloved of politicians in the late 1990s. There are lots of potential mixes in a mixed economy. All of them are trying to achieve the maximum output from the minimum input to the benefit of the greatest number of people. However, the devil is in the detail: who should make the decisions, where should the priorities be and what are the opportunity costs?

The focus of this chapter will be mainly on the behaviour of individuals. How do individuals make decisions? What influences those decisions? What does that mean for delivery of a service at the 'sharp end'?

Economics is a child of the age in which it was born. Its first ideas were developed in Europe in the period from 1750 to 1850. To this day it still bears the marks of ideas born in the Age of Enlightenment and a more mechanical approach to gathering knowledge. We study human behaviour when individuals make choices limited by lack of resources. This sounds fine but gets very complicated in the real world. So to make the analysis easier, underlying assumptions are made. We assume that individuals make decisions that are goal driven rather random. Also, the goals that drive these decisions remain roughly the same over time. Individual goals can change but not too rapidly; it would only complicate the analysis. We also assume that individuals are 'rational' in the process they go through when making any decision. I know you don't have to say it: I have a twelve-year-old daughter whose behaviour on any shopping trip challenges this assumption! The 'economic rational' person is the cornerstone of much theorising in economics and quite a bit in politics as well.

So what does 'economically rational' mean? It means people act consistently over time. They act to get the best satisfaction ('utility' in economic jargon) from what they consume. It makes no moral judgement on the things people consume. It can mean that some consumers appear to act in an apparently irrational way, for example putting their own life at risk by donating a kidney to a loved one. It may mean that some consumers stop or lower their own consumption to allow someone else to consume more: parents reduce their own consumption to send children through education, or more altruistically, people donate to developing countries to help someone they do not know and will never meet. All of this is 'rational' economic behaviour. The 'utility' the consumer gets from buying a goat for a hill farmer in Bolivia is greater than buying the goat (or something else) for themselves. They are still maximising their satisfaction, maximising their 'utility'.

This 'rationality' may still mean consumers are disappointed when they consume. The holiday that does not live up to the brochure description or the deodorant that does less for your sex life than the advertising says can be disappointing. However, the consumer was still trying to maximise utility. They failed to do this because of ignorance or a lack of information rather than a descent into irrationality. So economic rationality does not automatically mean everyone becomes a consumer hedonist. You do not need to be driven only by consumption to be an economically rational individual. The assumption of economic rationality may not be perfect but it gives us some insight into a process where we only partially understand what is going on and, so far, have identified some, but not all, of the factors involved.

So we have a set of assumptions in place to help us explain behaviour. What does the theory say should happen? The theory predicts two very different types of behaviour from what are two distinct groups of 'players' in this particular game. On the one side is the 'consumer': the person who ends up using whatever it is we are looking at. The 'consumer' is more often than not also the 'buyer' of the service or service. Beware though: there is a difference in the behaviour of a 'consumer' and of a 'buyer'. Currently in the NHS, buyers (healthcare 'commissioners') are not the same as consumers of healthcare (the patients). Unless I say otherwise, I assume the 'consumer' and the 'buyer' are the same person. This is yet another simplifying assumption. On the other side is the supplier. The supplier is the person or group of people who provide the service so the consumer can use it.

Both groups share some common behaviour. Both groups will carry on doing things for as long as they gain something from doing it. For both, the more they consume (or supply) the greater their gain ('the higher their total utility' in the jargon of economics). However as they consume (or supply) more, the increase in utility each new unit brings gets smaller and smaller gains (their marginal utility falls, in the jargon). Think cream cakes! The first cream cake is pretty wonderful. The second cream cake is still pretty good but is not quite as wonderful as the first. Each cake eaten at a single sitting becomes less and less pleasurable. Pausing for a day or two to allow the guilt to go down doesn't count. Usually consumers carry on consuming more of a service until they can see no more benefit in doing so (until their marginal utility becomes zero). The same is true of suppliers.

Consumers' behaviour

This process is also true of consumers of health services. People will continue to use health services for as long as *they perceive* they get some benefit (utility) for so doing. I emphasis their perception deliberately. It is what the consumer believes that is important to determining consumer behaviour. The supplier may think that the service they supply will not work, or is only going to be partially successful, or is a waste of scarce resources or even that it is a wonderful cure for all problems. What the supplier believes is immaterial, unless it is used to alter the consumer's perception. *In extremis* parents will still want to 'consume' health services for a child suffering from a terminal illness, even if this prolongs life by no more than a few weeks. The consumers perceive they get some benefit.

This is reflected in the comments in some of the examples in Part II. In Chapter 2, Katherine's mother says 'I was back and forward to the GP for months ... they kept telling me that I was a paranoid mother.' She clearly carries on consuming the service because she seeks to gain something, some utility, from the process. The actual delivery may not be what she wants. Certainly this supplier does not share this consumer's view of what is going on or what is needed, but the consumer carries on wanting to consume. Similarly in Chapter 4, the parent of Thomas states 'Everything we have needed for Thomas hasn't been there and what we have got for him we have had to push for.'

Returning to less extreme circumstances, consumers will consume for as long as their perceived gains in utility are greater than the costs of consuming. Usually in most markets these 'costs' are represented by the market price the consumer has to pay to get the service. In the UK, for the last 50 or so years, this has not been the case in much of the market for health services.

In those parts of healthcare that are 'free at the point of delivery' there is no obvious market price to the consumer. Therefore consumers, all acting logically, will continue to consume more and more of any particular health service until the perceived utility they get from that service reaches a peak (that is, until their marginal utility reaches zero). This position is bound to involve a higher level of consumption than the level that would apply with any form of market price. The higher the market price, the earlier the individual consumer will have felt that enough is enough and they are paying more for a service than they are benefiting from it. The higher the market price, the lower the level of consumption. The lower the market price, the higher the level of consumption of that service or services. In many parts of the UK health service market, the consumer's perception is 'it is free, so we will use it'.

Clearly the real world of UK healthcare isn't quite as baldly simple as that. Consumers do have costs other than the market price when trying to consume a service. Another idea from the dawn of economics is that of 'opportunity cost'. This is the cost of whatever the consumer has to give up, to consume the service in question. Thinking cream cakes again, the consumer might have given up the chance of a cup of coffee and a sandwich to buy a cream cake instead. If I take my child to therapy I will have to give up the chance of going shopping or to the pub. There is always some sort of resource involved. At the very least, time is a discrete, finite and non-renewable resource that has to be given up to do (consume) something else. To consume even a 'free' service the consumer has to give up their time. Often in consuming 'free' services there are other things (e.g. transport) that have to be consumed at the same time as the 'free' service. These 'complementary services' (economic jargon strikes again) also have a cost to the consumers. The higher the cost of these complementary services, the less of the 'free' service will be consumed.

Even for 'free services' consumers will continue consuming only up to the point where their utility from that service is greater than their 'opportunity cost'. For example, say providing a service involves the consumer in a 100-mile round trip by road and setting aside at least half a working day to do so. Even though the service itself is 'free at the point of delivery' the consumer will only consume if the perceived benefit outweighs the 'costs' of the 100-mile round trip and the half day of missed work (or pleasure). The greater the opportunity cost, the lower the consumption.

The price of the service is not the only factor influencing consumption. The price of any alternative (if there is one) will alter consumption of the service. If a cheap effective alternative appears, consumers will switch from the original service into the new, cheaper alternative. If the price of that alternative then rises, consumption of the original service will begin to rise in proportion to the increase in the price of the alternative service. Consumers switch back to make the most 'utility' from their limited available resources.

There is a third type of price that will alter consumption. If a second good or service has to be consumed with the original service, then the price of the second service will alter consumption of the first. Say a health service involves the purchase of pills and potions by the 'consumer'. If the price of those pills and potions rises, then the take-up of the original health service will fall. The size of this impact clearly depends on how significant the prices of the pills and potions are in relation to the utility gained from the original health service. If the prices of the pills and potions are low and the benefit of the health service high, then quite large rises in the prices of the pills and potions will have very little effect on the take-up of the original health service.

As incomes rise, people consume more of most services, including health care. Indeed some forms of health service (like cosmetic surgery) are considered a 'luxury good' by economists. A luxury good means that as income rises, the consumer increases their consumption of the good concerned at a faster rate than their increase in income. A common measure of personal income in the UK is gross domestic product per head. If you remove the effects of inflation, this measure shows average personal income has risen from £13,127 per annum in 1996 to £19,547 in 2004.[3] Average personal income has risen, so the desire to consume health services should also have risen, regardless of any changes in the size of the UK population. Of course the UK population has also been growing during the same period. The total population was 58,164,000 in 1996 and by 2003 rose to 59,554,000.[3] The population will continue to grow for the next decade. This also adds further to the quantity of health services consumed.

Supplier's behaviour

So how does this look from the supplier's point of view? One of the first questions to ask is who is 'the supplier'? Is it the individual practitioner actually in contact with the patients? Is it the manager who decides which practitioner goes where and what resources are allocated? Is it the organisation providing the money to pay for all this activity? In economic terms 'the supplier' will be the individual or group who takes the decisions on what is to be done, by whom and at what cost.

'The supplier' is the one with the freedom to choose to stop doing what they are doing and do something completely different, or to change the way they deliver a particular service. It is this ability to make the significant decisions that critically distinguishes a 'supplier' from others. In the UK healthcare market the 'supplier' is often not one single person but a mixture of various roles, sometimes in different organisations. The key to understanding is to distinguish the service provider from the 'supplier' of the service. The service provider in current NHS jargon is not usually the 'supplier' of economic theory.

In classic economic market system theory, the assumption is that a supplier is seeking to make the most profit they can. Therefore the key driver of a supplier's behaviour is the difference between the costs of providing a service and the price at which that same service can be sold to a consumer. The greater the difference between the costs of production and the selling price, the greater the profit per unit for the supplier. There are two behaviours to get the maximum profit: increase the price as high as the supplier can 'get away with' or reduce the costs of production to as low as possible while providing an 'adequate' standard of product for the customer. Clearly the real world of a profit maximiser is a combination of both behaviours in varying degrees. In classic theory, if the costs of production are greater than the price at which the service can be sold, then the supplier will not enter the market in the first place. Price acts as the key signal for the supplier in deciding what to do and how much resource to commit to doing it. In the NHS this key signal is missing. There is no price to link buyer perceptions to supplier resource use. Therefore the NHS is driven to substitute more complex and inherently less efficient ways of linking buyer perception and supplier resource decisions.

Are suppliers in the UK health market seeking to make the most profit they can? Evidence of their behaviour suggests not. They may be seeking to create the largest service or service the greatest number of clients or meet the targets imposed by central government. Very few suppliers in the UK health market appear to be attempting to maximise their profit. What does this mean for the use of resources and rationing? Classic economic analysis says that in these circumstances both the scale of output and the individual price of the particular service will be greater than the optimum for the economy as a whole. Also, the supplier will be providing this service at an average cost above the absolute minimum average cost that could be achieved if the market were left alone. All of this means that more physical resources are switched to this service and at a cost that is greater than that which is most efficient for the economy as a whole.

So what on earth is happening in the health market where the service is 'free at the point of delivery'? Any market for a service where the supplier has to give the service away for free ought not to have anyone prepared to supply into it. That is not the case in the UK health market, so what is going on?

In this market those who consume the service do not pay the supplier. The supplier is rewarded by an agency acting on behalf of central government. Central government is by its very nature a bureaucratic organisation. 'Bureaucratic' is used in the sense defined by Max Weber, the German sociologist. Weber identified bureaucracy as: 'A hierarchical structure of roles, with job holders appointed by merit and subject to rules, with an expectation of impartial behaviour' (Weber 1947).

The people who pay for the 'free' service are all those who pay UK taxes (value added tax, excise duty, income tax, corporation tax). These people do not have a direct influence over how their money is used. Predominately, in the UK, central government decides how this money is to be used. The drawback with this method is that there is no signalling method from client to supplier. In a market system, price and the interaction of supply and demand provide these signals. Even in real world markets with many faults and failings, these signals are still evident. The signals do not exist at all in a command system, free at the point of delivery.

So what does this mean for the front-line practitioner? Demand for services will always be greater than the resources you have available to provide that service. Therefore two types of behaviour are key to the role. The first is to strive constantly to deliver more with the resources you do have available. The increase in outcomes achieves the 'productive efficiency' of economic theory. The second behaviour is to create substitute mechanisms that mimic the feedback from clients provided by price and demand in an open market. Only by doing this will decisions on who gets scare resources, how much each client gets or who 'most deserves' the resources, match the perceptions of the clients themselves. The ideal solution is to get the client to make these decisions themselves rather than leave it to a supplier, no matter how well intentioned the supplier.

Where clients feel themselves directly involved in decision making their perceptions of service levels are significantly higher. Take the example of the children's palliative care specialist nurse in Chapter 5. The nurse felt that she had wrongly prioritised the order of her visits. Yet the family of the child:

> did not appear to share this. They expressed only gratitude that I had visited as they had requested . . . Written feedback from them since his death has confirmed that whilst the speed of his death had shocked them, they are positive about the peacefulness of his death and feel they were well supported in caring for their son at home.

> (p. 28)

The significance of a client's opportunity costs and utility perceptions can be seen in the use of triage in speech and language therapy (Chapter 7). Parents were encouraged to initiate first contact after a letter acknowledging receipt of referral was sent to them.

> The advantage of encouraging parents to initiate the contact and centralise the booking was that parents could then choose a clinic and a time that was convenient from the full range of options including short notice cancellations.

A local audit revealed that 85 per cent of parents responded to the letter asking them to make contact.

(p. 36)

From the service provider's viewpoint, 'the effect on attendance was dramatic' (p. 37). This shows consumer's opportunity cost and utility theory in action.

In a classic market system, if demand for a service was greater than supply, the price of that service would go up. In a service 'free at the point of delivery' that option is not available. So we constantly see 'Demand . . . outstrips their supply . . . waiting lists for SLT have tended to be long in many areas of the UK . . . (even though) . . . Waiting for therapy may be very stressful for parents and causes concern to practitioners and managers' (p. 35).

In an open market, new suppliers would be drawn in by the opportunities and apparent rewards. The new suppliers (and the existing ones) would all be trying to get the maximum profit they possibly can by providing the maximum quantity of a service that the consumers want, at a quality standard consumers are prepared to pay for and at a price consumers are willing to pay.

This all takes time to achieve. Some suppliers get it wrong. Suppliers cease to exist, some through bankruptcy, some by leaving the market when the going gets tough, some because they see better pickings elsewhere. This 'churning' of suppliers is a critical part of the quasi-biological workings of the market system. The whole process of allocating resources and establishing priorities in a market has a very Darwinian feel to it. However for this Darwinian economics to work properly, certain things have to be in place.

The process takes time. The market needs time to work through all the cause and effect relationships. Some reactions are a lot quicker than others. Therefore the market system is not going to prioritise instantly. The market system also may not prioritise well during the period when the adjustments are working through. In the end the priorities set should be the 'best' possible solution, the most economically efficient solution in the jargon, providing nothing else changes. Any new change, say in technology or cost of resources, should trigger a new bout of adjustments.

The process involves the 'birth' and 'death' of suppliers. It is an integral part of the efficiency in prioritising achieved by a market. New entrants come in and old hands leave a market. Suppliers have to come and go, to enter and leave the market. Increasing the efficiency with which we prioritise options is just one form of developing our knowledge. In the late 1980s Marsh investigated how organisations 'learnt' and concluded, 'The development of knowledge may depend on maintaining an influx of the naïve and the ignorant . . . competitive victory does not reliably go to the properly educated' (Marsh, 1991).

The strength and efficiency of the market-led process comes from giving consumers and suppliers the freedom to make mistakes. Surowiecki concludes that the best decisions are reached by generating as diverse a set of possible solutions in the first place. Then the next step is to create as diverse a group of decision makers as possible to make any decisions needed. These decision takers need

2   If you wish to explore more of the subject a good starting point is a general textbook such as John Sloman's *Economics* (2006) (FT/Prentice Hall).
3   Source: Office of National Statistics, National Income Blue Book 2005 (www.ons.gov. uk).
4   The Wanless Report (February 2004) *Securing Good Health for the Whole Population*. London: HMSO.

References

Department of Health (2005) *Creating a Patient-led NHS – Delivering the NHS Improvement Plan*. London: HMSO.

Department of Health (2006) *Our Health, our Care, our Say: A New Direction for Community Services*. London: HMSO White Paper.

Marsh, J.G. (1991) 'Exploration and Exploitation in Organisational Learning', *Organisational Science* **2**: 71–87.

Page, S. and Hong, L. (2001) 'Problem Solving by Heterogeneous Agents', *Journal of Economic Theory* **97**: 123–63.

Surowiecki, J. (2004) *The Wisdom of Crowds*. Boston: Little, Brown.

Weber, M. (1947) *Theory of Social and Economic Organisation* (trans. A. M. Henderson and T. Parsons) New York: The Free Press.

Weber, M. (1921) *Theory of Social and Economic Organisation*. New York: The Free Press.

Chapter 12

Prioritisation

An educationist's perspective

Geoff Lindsay

Introduction

Prioritisation acknowledges upfront the fact that resources are inadequate and so must be managed effectively. This is a truism but is an uncomfortable statement as it can be interpreted in terms of fault. It also reflects the reality of a welfare model of provision as opposed to a free market. In the latter, resources are accessed primarily by ability to pay, or to exert sufficient alternative influence: the needs of a child are effectively irrelevant.

The current position in the UK and many other countries in the West is that there are two significant societal changes occurring in parallel against which prioritisation must be considered. First, there is a change from primarily a welfare model to an increased use of markets (see Chapter 11). Currently we have a mixed economy, albeit heavily weighted to state provision, but where the influence of the state has diminished and is likely to continue to diminish. The 'third way' (Giddens 1998) is a deliberate policy of the present government and is likely to continue in essence under any other party for the foreseeable future.

The second change concerns consumerism and the move from the state and its representatives making decisions, to the consumer of education and health services being recognised either as having a rightful role as a partner, co-decision maker, or even as being the person who makes decisions. Of particular note is the fundamental change in the legal rights of parents following the Education Act 1981 and subsequent revisions which built on the recommendations of the Warnock Committee (Department for Education and Science 1978) that parents should be partners. Since that time, the role of parents in decision making has increased dramatically, and the need to support professionals in working with parents has been recognised (Wolfendale 2002).

It is important to recognise that these two issues are distinct but interact. For example, consumerism brings with it more power for the individual compared with the state and this may, in a mixed economy, be used to access services outside the state system. The present government has encouraged this and indeed the most recent education White Paper (Department for Education and Skills 2005) has developed this thinking further, with proposals for independent schools to federate with local authority schools.

Prioritisation must be considered against this background. In the past, prioritisation was often operationalised by the simple model of the waiting list. This
was an example of professionals (or in some cases administrators acting by
default) determining service delivery, and hence prioritisation, within the state
system. The growth of a range of service providers, the threat of privatisation
of services and the growth of consumer power to demand action are all important
and real.

In this chapter I shall propose a systematic examination of the issues that affect
prioritisation, within a broad sociopolitical framework. The main reason for starting
with the latter has been to stress that prioritisation cannot be seen simply in terms
of factors relating to the individual needs of the child. Rather, this analysis proposes
a series of domains of factors, each of which must be considered. Also, and
consequently, these domains must be seen as acting together within a total system.
But first I shall consider how conflicts may arise between health and education in
their decision making.

Where conflicts may arise

Conflict between health and education may arise at different levels, e.g. between
policy makers and practitioners. It is possible to locate the types of problems at
these different levels but with recognition that there is overlap.

Practitioner level

The first example concerns conceptualisation. A national study of educational
provision for children with specific speech and language difficulties identified
significant differences in approaches by speech and language therapists (SLTs)
and educationists (Dockrell et al. 2006; Lindsay et al. 2005). The former tended to
use diagnostic approaches, which the latter eschewed. While both groups were
concerned to identify the children's needs, the SLTs were also concerned to
diagnose the type of problem or disorder. Hence, in practice, conflicts can occur over
the salience of diagnostic categories and their usefulness. This has been exemplified
by the frequently confused debate over dyslexia (e.g. see Elliott 2005) and the
accompanying letters in *The Psychologist* (December, 2005). The essential issue is
that such developmental problems have no clear and objectively defined cut-offs
to aid a diagnostic approach and, equally important, research evidence may fail to
support the necessity to distinguish one group from another. Difficulties between
professionals using or rejecting diagnostic categories such as dyslexia and autistic
spectrum disorder are, essentially, unresolvable as they reflect paradigm differences
in conceptualisation.

The second area for dispute concerns intervention, particularly location. Faced
with a child with major speech and language difficulties, an SLT may seek a
placement in a special facility (special school or integrated resource/language unit)
where language can be addressed with expertise and relatively high resourcing.

An educationist such as an educational psychologist (EP), however, may seek a mainstream setting, taking a broader perspective of the child's total needs.

The third area is the use of assessment. Many EPs have reduced their use of standardised normative assessments while SLTs often find these useful. Conflict can occur if the SLT seeks a measure of non-verbal ability which the EP does not see as important. Fourth, practitioners may disagree about patterns of delivery, for example, over the implementation of contributions (e.g. the exact model, who is involved, who consults whom etc.) or a concern that too many professionals are acting as consultants – so, who is actually delivering?

In all of these examples, the issues concern differences of views or actions by one professional impacting on others. Disputes between other professionals can impact on teachers as well as between health professionals and teachers themselves.

Service level

Here disputes often involve either finance or service organisation and delivery. The former may concern the funding of SLTs, with recent developments in funding either jointly or by local authorities (Law *et al.* 2000). In the absence of formal arrangements, a trust may reduce service delivery to schools as it attempts to meet other priorities. This impacts on schools, who may be able to do little as they do not control the finance.

A second issue concerns overall policies, the most significant at present being inclusion. This may be seen positively in principle, but it raises challenges for professionals who must visit many locations rather than a few specialist facilities and who may consider the support provided in mainstream education does not match that available in a specialist setting.

Some degree of conflict may be inevitable as different services have different degrees of freedom regarding their own prioritisation of service delivery. Jointly determined prioritisation therefore poses specific additional challenges, and this can be further undermined if the issues considered here, such as different conceptualisations, are also in play.

A systematic view of decision making

The argument in this chapter is that a systematic analysis of decision making regarding prioritisation of services to children must take account of the following:

- child factors
- system factors
- the local and national sociopolitical context
- interaction of these three.

In addition it is proposed that the determination of any prioritisation system must also pay attention to how this system is agreed, and then how it is communicated.

Child factors

A number of child factors have been highlighted in Part II. I shall build upon these, but also discuss why they are important. The nature of the child's presenting needs will vary on a number of dimensions, and these will be of different relevance to the various professionals involved.

This dimension concerns, first, the relevance of the type of problem to the professional. This may not always be apparent on first presentation but must be taken into account. For example, a child not attending school may or may not be within the province of an education welfare officer. In many cases this is clear, for example when absence can reasonably be attributed to an acute illness, but often it is not. Categorisation of absence into authorised and unauthorised partly addresses the issue of type, but these are not absolute categories; indeed the type of absence accepted as authorised has changed recently.

Similarly, determining whether a child with an emotional problem should be seen by an EP or clinical psychologist is not straightforward; or whether a child with language and literacy difficulties should be seen by an SLT, psychologist or a special education needs (SEN) specialist.

These problems arise for two main reasons. First, there may, and often is (Rutter *et al.* 1970) more than one presenting significant issue. Second, there is a question of the order in which different professionals might be engaged so as to optimise the information gained and passed on, and the determination of whether to intervene and, if so, how.

Age

Age is often viewed as a key domain: the younger the better. Teachers will frequently argue that a child should be seen early in their school, or should have been seen earlier than now. This is based upon a linear view of development; a child presenting problems now will continue to do so unless intervention occurs. As such it ignores the phenomena of differential trajectories and evidence, both of spontaneous remission, where a child improves without intervention, and evidence of children moving in and out of 'at risk' or 'problem' categories.

Furthermore, it may not be the case that a suitable intervention is available for the age of the child. For example, there has been much interest since the 1970s in preventing reading difficulties in children. Attempts to identify children as 'at risk' of failing to develop competent reading have not proven successful, because of the large number of inaccurate identifications found in early screening programmes (Lindsay and Wedell 1982).

However, despite these caveats, age is certainly an important factor and should be considered in every case, but this must be balanced against these other factors.

Severity

Problems differ in severity on several dimensions. Any particular problem may vary within its domain. This is a technical question of identifying the degree of severity. However, in cases where there are several problem dimensions the judgement becomes more complex. For example, the growth in the popularity of the construct autistic spectrum disorder has fundamentally changed the conceptualisation of 'autism'. When autism was the term of choice, the concern was with a very low incidence group of children. The use of autistic spectrum disorder multiplies considerably the number of children as it includes a wider range of severity, and this is applied to each of the three dimensions of importance in this condition. Hence, for example, a child might be identified on the basis of significant concern on one dimension, but whose development on the other two is barely within the range of relevance. What is effectively a change in definition (albeit with different terms) has been a major factor in the apparent increase in 'autism' according to a national study of local authorities' SEN officers and heads of speech and language therapy services (Dockrell *et al*. 2006).

Consideration of severity must also compare different types of difficulty. For example, in Chapter 5 Tara Kerr-Elliott and Nicola Eaton discuss a dying child and the question of prioritisation of actions. This is an extreme case, but raises both the technical questions discussed so far, and below, and the emotional dimension. However rational the prioritisation system, there may be occasions when an emotionally based decision is made. If one extrapolates backwards it is arguable that many decisions will have varying degrees of emotional as well as rational causation. If this is so we must be aware of this propensity in general and examine its operation and pertinence in any specific case.

Hence, while severity is a sound factor to govern prioritisation, I would argue that it is not straightforward. Both evidential and emotional factors should be considered.

Efficacy

Implicit in the previous discussion is the question of efficacy – what works and how well? For example, even if a child's presenting problem is high on other dimensions requiring high prioritisation, should this occur if we have no good evidence that what we are likely to do will have any positive benefit? This requires a broad view of benefit – emotional support may be very important even if nothing to address the problem *per se* is available. But we must also be aware that when undertaking one action we prevent another, so resources are used that could have been deployed where there is a higher chance of success.

This dimension requires an up-to-date awareness of the evidence for the effectiveness of alternative actions, whether for assessment of or intervention with a child.

Personal skills and preferences

Any qualified professional will be trained in their discipline to an agreed set of standards but as they work, competence profiles may diverge. There may continue to be a central core of common work, but different staff take on different quasi-specialist roles. Sometimes these are structurally related (e.g. child *vs* adult services) but often they reflect local circumstances (e.g. working with children for whom English is an additional language) or personal 'preference' (e.g. following a particular type of continuing professional development). This can be most clearly seen in services such as educational psychology where there is both a wide range of possible presenting issues and a degree of freedom to decide where to put one's energies. Many services have addressed this by matching individual skills with service needs (see below) but the 'unspoken' factor is that of preference, whether conscious or not.

For example, a discussion in the Sheffield Psychology Service when I was Principal addressed the question: why do referral roles for adolescents threatening suicide vary? The working hypothesis was that some EPs were interested and hence 'attracted' such referrals. Elaboration of this debate identified other types of problem with apparently similar differential patterns of referral not obviously linked to absolute need.

The reason for raising this is not to suggest this is inappropriate behaviour. First, it is put forward as a characteristic of human systems which, however rational the decision making, will include a degree of the personal. Second, there is a benefit in recognising and responding to this factor by matching it with expertise. So, such preferences can be built upon to develop quasi-specialist or specialist roles.

Prioritisation therefore needs to take account of the skills available and be organised to optimise their use. A generic service, with all professionals offering the same service, may be an appropriate first model of provision, but a second-order specialist/quasi-specialist function responding to individuals' strengths is also helpful.

Underlying this discussion is an ethical question regarding competence. While all qualified practitioners in a particular role are expected to have the necessary competencies for the core job, serendipitous variation by personal whim is of questionable relevance, while planned optimisation of enhanced competence is ethical.

System factors

In this section I shall address the characteristics and needs of the system in which the prioritisation must occur. This approach to systems analysis and understanding is necessary to provide a full context of decision making. For example, a recent study of 'good practice' for children with specific speech and language difficulties examined the operation of the total system from the top (policy making by the local authorities and trusts) through the implementation of policy at structural level (e.g. deployment of SLTs, EPs etc.; use of language units/integrated resources and mainstream support) down to what actually happens to the child (the individual and joint practice of SLTs, EPs, teachers, teaching assistants, and special educational needs co-ordinators (SENCOs)); and how parents relate to each of these levels (Dockrell 2005; Lindsay 2005). The essence of this study was to demonstrate that good practice could be identified at each level but that for successful implementation, attention needed to be paid to the interaction of each element of this total system.

Resources

Availability of resources should not affect the type of prioritisation as such; however strong the resource base, decisions will still be required. Rather, levels of resources will sharpen up thinking about the types of work to undertake. Variation in levels of resources may affect not just a model of prioritisation where, for example, a waiting time doubles as resources are halved. Rather, it may lead to a debate about *whether* to undertake certain work at all, and the relative resources to allocate to any type of work. As services have developed and grown, it is tempting to consider more of the same when extra provision is made, but there is benefit in rethinking major categories of work with consequent major system changes. An example is the introduction of a triage system described by Caroline Pickstone in Chapter 7.

Child-based and other work

Many healthcare professionals have the individual child as their primary focus, but this approach has been challenged over recent years, for example with the development of a consultancy model by SLTs. These developments in health reflect development in the 1970s and 1980s within educational psychology. As the profession expanded following the Summerfield Report (Department for Education and Science 1968) many services were unable to deal with increasing numbers of children. Prioritisation was often implemented by the waiting list with all its attendant limitation.

Some services recognised that the current way of working would only lead to increasing numbers of referrals even if the profession were increased by 200–300 per cent or more, as there was so much unmet perceived need. They took a lateral move and decided to focus some of their energies on the school system rather than the child. For example, rather than assessing a series of poor readers and making recommendations to teachers, they ran consultation or in-service education (Inset) programmes. This 'systems work' proved popular with EPs and also with schools, a marked and radical departure from referral-driven individual work (Gillham 1978; Leadbetter,2004; Lindsay and Miller 1991; Stoker 1999). Training aims for EPs reflected these developments and added systems work to that of individual child-based practice. This practice was endorsed by a recent government review of the profession (Department for Education and Employment 2000).

This practice was taken up by other services including SEN support services and SLTs (Law *et al.* 2000) so that now it is a common strand across services. The issue for prioritisation is two-fold at service level. First, the relative proportion of resources to be allocated to this area of work must be balanced by individual child work. Second, resource allocation and prioritisation must be decided within this category, just as within child-based work. Evidence of effectiveness and consumer desire will affect these decisions although it is difficult to achieve firm evidentially based decisions. The evidence to support practice A or practice B may not be readily available, and indeed is often not possible to achieve simply as 'hard' evidence. For example, choosing whether to prioritise practice which will enhance the situation of all poor readers compared with that of a subgroup of children with English as an additional language includes value judgement in addition to any evidence of relative effectiveness.

Systems work must also be considered on other dimensions. For example, some is intended specifically to be preventative, e.g. through skilling front-line workers. Other work provides a more cost-effective delivery of an assessment or intervention service. It is, however, important to be clear of the purpose and anticipated benefits. In any case, evaluation of these practices should then be examined. For example, within SEN support, the favoured philosophy within education has moved increasingly to inclusive education. This has largely been driven by a concern for children's rights but I have argued elsewhere that evidence for efficacy is far from clear (Lindsay 2003). One outcome of inclusion has been the increasing use of teaching assistants (TAs) to work with individual children: put crudely, the model adopted is that a statement is equated with a number of hours of TA time, rather than a more extended series of specific elements of support. This approach has financial (and hence administrative) simplicity but takes little note of TA expertise or the specific needs of the child. There is also a lack of evidence for its effectiveness.

Formula-driven prioritisation

How, then, should decisions of service allocation of resources be made? Several factors are relevant, including overall levels of resources, especially staff; qualified professionals and assistants; and basic expertise and advanced skills. Two other approaches have been used, in addition, with success.

As described by Caroline Pickstone in Chapter 7, triage has been an effective means of overcoming a referral-driven, waiting-list based system. It allows early action, leading to decisions of child priorities determined by factors such as those described above.

A second approach, developed by EP services and others in education, is to allocate resources, in part, by use of general proxy measures. Many psycho-educational difficulties are correlated with social disadvantage so systems of allocation have been developed based on measures of this (typically, free-school-meals entitlement). Usually the school is taken as the unit of measurement. For example, the system I developed with colleagues in the Sheffield Psychological Service in the early 1990s allocated resources to schools on the basis of numbers on roll multiplied by a social disadvantage factor from 1 to 2, i.e. highly disadvantaged schools could receive up to twice as much EP time as a same-sized school with highly socially advantaged pupils. In addition, separate factors were built in to address special schools and systems work.

It is important to stress that this model uses the school as a proxy to aid the resource allocation. The service is provided to the school and its community, i.e. its pupils and their parents. This point is important as it is a prioritisation of overall resources, not a prioritisation of individual decisions. For example, in this model an allocation of, say, 5 days of EP time to the school must be used for all work arising in the area, including referrals from parents, GPs, SLTs and other professionals. There is still a need to prioritise within the five days and care is necessary to ensure that the school's priorities are judged against those of others.

Prioritisation decisions must then be made at a second level, i.e. the work arising from this area, not just that identified by the school. Often this is determined by the EP in collaboration with the SENCO and/or other professionals Attempts to have large-scale multidisciplinary meetings for this purpose have, in my experience, been very problematic. For example, getting everyone together is difficult in itself and is wasteful if not every child needs consideration by every professional.

This approach is also neutral on the question of action. For example, the time allocation may be used for individual work, for consultation provided to the teachers and/or parents by an individual professional or to joint consultation, assessment or intervention by two or more professionals. The main characteristic is to allocate firstly by general assessment of need and refined at the second level to prioritise actions.

The sociopolitical context

What is less easy to define is the determination of prioritisation by 'political' influence. The hard version of this concerns the pressure brought to bear to prioritise a child because a councillor or member of parliament (MP) has taken an interest. A second variant concerns media interest in a child, and pressure brought by senior management to act swiftly to avoid embarrassment to the organisation rather than because the child's needs demand such prioritisation. The third variant concerns parental pressure. This is more subtle and problematic. Some parents have, or develop, very effective abilities to put maximum pressure on professionals and service managers, e.g. to prioritise actions or the type of outcome. On the other hand, many parents have low levels of such awareness and skill, and may even be properly described as disempowered.

It is easy to state that any such pressures should be ignored, and that a professional judgement should be made simply on the child's needs. It can be more difficult to implement. Nevertheless, this must be the case if the professional and service are to behave ethically.

Any variant away from this must be weighed carefully in terms of the disadvantage to other children and parents. This may not be straightforward. It may be judged that the time necessary to resist what is seen as inappropriate pressure, perhaps ending in a Special Educational Needs and Disability Tribunal, provides more disadvantage to other children in terms of wasted professional time than does complying. These are fine judgements. In any case, the main aim should be to avoid such situations occurring and, indeed, this should also be built into service prioritisation, for example through the work of the head of service as well as any individual practitioner. In my experience, almost all parents, and indeed councillors and MPs, who engage in this behaviour do so for what they regard as the right reasons, not to be self-seeking or malicious. A priority, therefore, is to optimise parents' and politicians' understanding of the service and the standards to which it operates to avoid such problems arising if at all possible.

Interaction

I have addressed a series of factors from three domains: child, service and political context. Implicit in the previous discussion is the need to consider these in interaction. For example, consideration of an 'enquiry' from an MP cannot be viewed simply as unwarranted interference but should also take into account the nature of the child's problems.

Similarly, and as indicated in the discussion of workload allocation, prioritisation must occur both within and between different aspects of work. The main example given here has been child-based compared with systems-based practice. This deserves a further discussion to exemplify the point. I have argued that a number of services have moved away from an emphasis on child-based work exclusively to one of working at a systems level. In this I have not discussed the role of the family, which may also be seen as a system including the child, and interaction with other systems such as the school. Hence, practice must also consider engagement with the family, which may take several forms. First, there is the right of parents to be involved in providing knowledge of the child, and to contribute to decision making. This does not imply 'the parent (mother) knows best', a rather unfortunate, glib statement that is often heard from professionals. Certainly parents have unique knowledge which must be valued, but this complements the knowledge and skills of professionals. This is the essence of effective partnership.

Second, parents may take a significant role in intervention (or assessment), e.g. running a programme at home supported by a professional. Third, the family system may require help beyond that of the individual child. Finally, parents can contribute to the system, from school to local or national policy and thereby beyond their own child to the population of children of concern. Hence, when discussing prioritisation with respect to parents, it is also important to consider these different roles and tasks, both of and for parents.

Communication and dissemination

Finally, prioritisation will be considered as a topic to be agreed and then disseminated. The means to decide the prioritisation also requires careful attention. The key players will be the service members themselves, especially the head of service or a delegated leader of this project. These are the experts. But there is much to be gained, both practically and politically, in working with others. One method is to survey opinion. This was a method I undertook when leading on a prioritisation system for the Sheffield Psychological Service. A survey of headteachers clearly showed that, in general, they were relatively satisfied with quality but not quantity, and they had clear views on a range of practices they valued (Lindsay 1991). This fed into a formal process of developing a model which was tested within the service, with a representative group of headteachers, and then presented to all headteachers in the city.

It is not suggested that this is always needed; the need here was magnified by the possibility of delegation of funding to schools. Nevertheless, the new system was welcomed: it was accepted that no prioritisation system could be perfect, but this was rational and likely to be fit for purpose. A second survey two years later confirmed its success, with marked improvements in ratings (Lindsay 1995). What is of general relevance is the need to involve stakeholders in the determination of the prioritisation system; to undertake a careful dissemination process which was interactive not simply informative; and then to evaluate the system in practice.

This approach must also take account of the interaction of the service system with other systems. As health and education have moved increasingly together, and with the 'Every Child Matters' agenda underway, there is even greater need for systems not only to talk to each other, but also to be developed in collaboration with each other. On the other hand, this must not lead to inaction as the perceived enormity of the task weighs heavily on all involved. There is a clear role here for action at several levels.

1. Initial training for all relevant professions must address prioritisation and I would argue this be done from a systems perspective.
2. The service must set down clear policies for general prioritisation decisions.
3. Each practitioner must individually consider prioritisation of their own work within the service framework.

Examples within this book demonstrate both that practitioners are engaged in such reflections and that this is not always easy. I therefore end with stressing that there is unlikely ever to be a 'perfect' system. What we can do is optimise a system's fitness for purpose by careful, rational analysis. This must then be tempered by a recognition that human systems, particularly those dealing with the vulnerable, the disadvantaged and those living with varying physical and psychological problems, must also take account of human emotions. Finally, as with conventions of ethical behaviour, we must acknowledge that however well developed the model and protocols, dilemmas will arise on occasion that require both careful reflections and analysis, and support from colleagues.

References

Department for Education and Employment (2000) *Educational Psychological Services (England): Current Role, Good Practice and Future Directions.* Nottingham: DfEE.

Department for Education and Skills (2005) *Higher Standards, Better Schools for All: More Choice for Parents and Pupils.* (Cm 6677). London: The Stationery Office.

Department for Education and Science (1968) *Psychologists in Education Services (The Summerfield Report).* London: HMSO.

Department for Education and Science (1978) *Special Educational Needs (The Warnock Report).* London: HMSO.

Dockrell, J.E., Lindsay, G., Letchford, C. and Mackie, C. (2006) Educational provision for children with specific speech and language difficulties: Perspectives of speech and language therapy managers. *International Journal of Language and Communication Disorders,* **41**: 423–40.

Dockrell, J. (2005) Systemic Approaches to Supporting Children with Specific Speech and Language Difficulties. Paper presented to the National Association of Professionals Concerned with Language Impairment in Children. University of Warwick, March

Elliott, J. (2005) 'Dyslexia: The debate continues', *The Psychologist,* **18**: 728–30.

Giddens, A. (1998). *The Third Way: The Renewal of Social Democracy.* London: Polity Press.

Gillham, W.E.C. (ed.) (1978) *Reconstructing Educational Psychology.* Beckenham: Croom Helm.

Law, J., Lindsay, G., Peacey, N., Gascoigne, M., Soloff, N., Radford, J. and Band, S. with Fitzgerald, L. (2000) *Provision for Children with Speech and Language Needs in England and Wales: Facilitating Communication Between Education and Health Services.* London: DfEE.

Leadbetter, J. (2004) 'The role of mediating artifacts in the work of educational psychologists during consultative conversations in schools', *Educational Review,* **56(2)**: 133–45.

Lindsay, G. (1991) 'The educational psychologist in the new era', in G. Lindsay and A. Miller (eds) *Psychological Services for Primary Schools.* London: Longman.

Lindsay, G. (1995) 'Sheffield Psychological Service – a quality case study', *Educational Psychology in Practice. Special issue: Management,* 39–43.

Lindsay, G. (2003) 'Inclusive education: A critical perspective', *British Journal of Special Education,* **30**: 3–12.

Lindsay, G. (2005). Barriers to good practice: where are we now? Paper presented to the National Association of Professionals Concerned with Language Impairment in Children. University of Warwick, March

Lindsay, G., Dockrell, J.E., Mackie, C. and Letchford, C. (2005) 'Local education authorities' approaches to provision for children with specific speech and language difficulties in England and Wales', *European Journal of Special Needs Education* **20**: 329–45.

Lindsay, G. and Miller, A. (eds) (1991) *Psychological Services for the Primary School.* Harlow: Longman.

Lindsay, G. and Wedell, K. (1982) 'The early identification of educationally "at risk" children: Revisited', *Journal of Learning Disabilities*, **15**: 212–17.

Rutter, M., Tizard, J. and Whitmore, K. (1970) *Education, Health and Behaviour*. Harlow: Longman.

Stoker, R. (1999) 'The sixth discipline of the learning organization – understanding the psychology of individual constructs and the organization', *Educational and Child Psychology*, **17(1)**: 76–85.

Wolfendale, S. (2002) *Parent Partnership Services for Special Educational Needs: Celebrations and Challenges*. London: David Fulton.

Part IV

Reflections on prioritisation

Chapter 13

Some answers questioned

Brian Petheram and Sue Roulstone

When originally conceived, the book was visualised as a tool for practitioners to support their thinking about prioritisation in child health. It was clear from the outset that there were no easy answers; indeed that is the major recurring theme throughout the literature on rationing: that provision of healthcare is complex and that simple solutions are unlikely to be forthcoming.

Producing this book has been like a research process in itself: the introductory chapter provided an opportunity to explore the background and existing literature. The second section, Part II, grounded the book in the real-life practices of everyday healthcare. Part III has provided a number of theoretical perspectives. We have used all of these chapters as stimuli to our own process of reflection on prioritisation, and as data for an exploration of the topic of prioritisation.

This chapter draws together some issues arising from and stimulated by the earlier chapters. We present them as a series of questions and discussions (rather than as questions and answers: as our title for this chapter suggests!) Unlike most research processes, you, as reader, have had access to our data in its entirety and are therefore in a position to come to your own conclusions about the key issues. It is highly likely that different issues may have struck a chord or been salient for different readers, which reflect their different context.

The introduction to this chapter and indeed to the whole book, accepts prioritisation as a fact of life. It pervades every level of healthcare from national decisions about what drugs or services are to be provided free at the point of delivery as part of the NHS, down to the individual practitioner managing their own workload. This book focuses on the latter, the micro level, examining the prioritisation decisions taken within particular services and by individual practitioners, rather than at a macro level of management across services and across the country.

Do we really have to prioritise?

One of the fundamental issues to arise concerns our interpretation of the context in which prioritisation decisions occur – how prioritisation is conceptualised and considered by an individual or a service. The contributors who have provided our examples demonstrate the amount of time and energy given to these decisions and the amount of anxiety they provoke, both in practitioners and in the people who use services. Practitioners blame themselves for their difficulties in managing time successfully and take work home in order to keep up with their workload. Words such as 'came to a head', 'compounded', 'dilemmas' speak of difficult situations that challenge the decision maker. Initially, the book itself was conceptualised as a problem-solving exercise, the aim being to support practitioners in finding solutions. Loughlin (Chapter 9) challenges us on a number of these and suggests we start our quest elsewhere, perhaps looking to the macro level and government to provide additional resources to support hard-pressed practitioners or perhaps at least to challenge our basic assumptions about the process under discussion. This seems to present us with a number of questions about that basic context.

- Is prioritisation inevitable?
- Will prioritisation decisions eventually solve problems of inadequate resources?
- Will prioritisation decisions provide a stop gap until the resourcing problems are resolved?
- Is there an alternative to prioritisation?
- Is it a 'winnable' situation? (see Chapter 9).

As indicated above, many writers on the subject of rationing or prioritisation talk of its inevitability. Weale (1995) for example asks the same question: 'Is rationing necessary?' He notes that system-wide change is difficult and infrequent and that this together with the increasing costs of healthcare, arising from technical innovations that become progressively more routine, results in a situation where rationing is unavoidable. Furthermore, all practitioners have to decide how to manage their day, which intervention to recommend, which child to see next. This minute-to-minute decision making clearly has implications for the overall management of resources in healthcare (Irvine and Donaldson 1995). Loughlin challenges us to think more radically and to 'call for a new game' in which the need to prioritise would itself be challenged. However, he too concludes that this is a long-term process which in the meantime requires us to survive the current system. The voices of our contributors reflect the common experience of a current healthcare service in which prioritisation becomes ever more evident. But this apparent all-pervasiveness of prioritisation becomes a challenge in itself: if it is so pervasive, is it possible to do anything about it? If change will take generations what should our response be?

As practitioners we should at least stop feeling guilty that we can't solve the problems. That doesn't mean we wash our hands and give up trying, but we don't need to beat ourselves up about it. What we sometimes regard as failures in the management of workloads are almost inevitable in the current system. Managing workloads and making decisions about how to use resources is and will be an ongoing issue for all healthcare workers for some time to come, maybe for generations.

Who takes responsibility?

So what are the options at this point? If the allocation of resources is an ongoing challenge, who takes responsibility for making these decisions? Should our hard-pressed practitioners be passing more decisions to their senior managers, letting the system deal with what are essentially systemic problems? However, as Weale (1995) comments, while it might ease the burden on front-line practitioners, if all prioritisation decisions are made at an institutional level, this can result in less sensible decisions for the individual.

The fundamental issue is that formal policies and procedures can only cope with the foreseeable, and healthcare practice is characterised by a variety of issues and factors that can arise in infinite combinations when treating a particular individual. To try to produce guidelines that attempt to allow for this would be impossibly complex and the resulting procedures would effectively be unusable. This is recognised by Dowie (2003) where he outlines a useful continuum of health-care situations from scientific experiments and randomised controlled trials to clinical judgements and maps them on to a matching continuum of analytic and judgemental approaches to decision making. This issue is picked up in the next section of this chapter when the 'programmability' of decisions is discussed. Catch-all prioritisation systems still have to be interpreted by the individual practitioner as they meet each child on their caseload and at each point throughout the management of a child: the decision making around the use of resources is not just about accessing services, but includes the ongoing management of a caseload.

Furthermore, we see clearly in the examples in Part II, the knock-on effects of prioritisation, which are often unplanned and even unpredicted. For example, changing how speech and language therapists work with preschool children has an impact on health-visiting services; unforeseen additional workloads for the palliative care team creates additional work for the community nurses; changing the type of physiotherapy service delivered creates a need for different kinds of physical resources. Prioritisation actions create changes in the behaviour of our clients and colleagues that impact upon the original prioritisation in ways that are not always clear when the decision is taken. Consider: a particular waiting list is prioritised; colleagues begin to refer to that service again, having previously counselled against referral because of long waiting lists; the funding directed at the service for prioritisation of this waiting list is unable to achieve the hoped-for impact because the number of referrals has grown substantially and the number on the waiting list have now doubled.

So decisions about prioritisation within a particular service obviously interact within that service and with other services and with other levels of prioritisation in the national system. The Rationing Agenda Group (New 1996) also asked who should be making this decision and set out a list of potential stakeholders, including the public, patients, families, user groups, healthcare professionals, managers, central and local government, the media, industry and the judiciary. They also discuss the difficulties of combining all these perspectives into one decision, and the number of stakeholders is clearly related to where the decision is being made, whether at macro or micro level. Within the evidence collected in this book, it seemed to be the tendency that, rather than being seen as an issue for the entire system to work on together, individual practitioners or services take on the 'problem solving' in isolation.

The parents at the start of the book were keen to be involved in the decision-making process on behalf of their children. They talk about having access to honest information and to practitioners themselves in order to be able to discuss inter-vention options. Yet the involvement of families in the prioritisation process appears to be less straightforward for practitioners. They recognise parents' concern and desire to do the best, but are struggling with how to balance the demands of parents who are able to articulate needs on behalf of their child with those who do not or cannot. The application of principles of partnership, which is the current expectation and aspiration of children's services generally, still seems elusive with respect to decisions about allocation of resources both for the individual family and at the service level.

There could be any number of reasons behind this – the speed at which decisions can be made in partnership, the personal ownership of the problem, a fear of the competing agendas of other stakeholders, to name but a few. Shickle (1997) points out some of the potential ethical issues relating to some of the expressed prefer-ences of the public (treating the young in preference to the elderly for example) that might give rise to concern when including a range of stakeholders in the process. However, decisions made in partnership are likely to be more acceptable to the wider group and therefore less likely to meet with opposition. Indeed, there is also the possibility (Chapter 11, p. 84) that constructive conflict is helpful in reaching difficult decisions, since the debate itself leads to a fuller exposure of the issues for consideration.

What methods are available for making prioritisation decisions?

The accounts in previous chapters indicate that a wide variety of methods are in use. This should not be regarded as a weakness or a 'problem', because prioritisa-tion takes place in a wide variety of contexts and circumstances. Thus it is unlikely that a single approach will be universally applicable. Any method or procedure is designed to address a particular situation and is therefore aimed at the predefined and the foreseen. However, there will always be issues that are unforeseen and different in detail from an original prioritisation procedure (the sudden death of the child described in Chapter 5 is a dramatic example). Therefore there will always be a place for professional judgement and discretion and all effective methods of prioritisation should leave some scope for this.

Prioritisation is essentially a decision-making process; Miers, in Chapter 10, provides an overview of the body of knowledge in the area of decision theory. Under this umbrella term there are varying accounts of the process of decision making, all of which have some resonances with the earlier chapters. For instance Croot (Chapter 6) describes a way of setting an overt framework to guide the allocation of resources, whereas Kerr-Elliott and Eaton (Chapter 5) describe a day in the life of a health professional which no policy is likely to account for! The original and classic theory is the rational model of decision making. This views decision making as a deliberative process that seeks to optimise performance relative to explicit criteria. A typical formulation is shown in Box 13.1.

Box 13.1

1. Define the problem.
2. Identify decision criteria.
3. Allocate weights to the criteria.
4. Develop possible courses of action.
5. Evaluate possible actions in relation to the criteria.
6. Choose action with maximum value.

This approach has been criticised, most notably by Herbert Simon (1977) as being dependent on unrealistic assumptions such as:

*   the problem is clear and unambiguous
*   criteria are agreed and can be ranked and weighted
*   all courses of action are both known and feasible in relation to cost, ethical and other constraints
*   there are unlimited resources available for the process of decision making itself.

Simon argues that in reality, decision makers exercise at best a bounded or limited rationality in that they use incomplete and simplified models that are evaluated against partially formulated criteria and where data to infill the above process are only partially available. If we are to be critically reflective about the decisions we make then it may be helpful to consider the extent to which these limitations apply to our own situations. How far are the criteria for prioritisation of children known and definable? Is the problem clear and unambiguous?

Pressures towards transparency and accountability in the NHS lead to a preference for rational models, as these are more easily explained and defended in those contexts. The most obvious example is the recent emphasis on evidence-based practice (EBP), the requirement to base one's practice on systematically acquired research evidence. Indeed, the mantra of EBP has been used as a counter to the need for rationing: the argument goes along the lines of 'if only we would use only proven interventions and stop doing those interventions where there is no evidence of effectiveness, then there would be no need for rationing'. This approach has met with some resistance, challenged in its conservative form as inappropriate to some groups, impossible to implement because of the complexities of applying and interpreting evidence collected in a group context to the care of individuals (Burton & Chapman 2004; Rycroft-Malone *et al.* 2004; van der Gaag *et al.* 2003). It is certainly unlikely that all aspects of practice will ever be covered by research evidence, particularly when the funding of research is, in itself, not an entirely neutral or evidence-based process (see for example Chard 2005). Consider also the complexity of the children whose stories were told in Part II. Some proponents of EBP recognise that the blind application of evidence is inappropriate and include notions of expertise and professional judgement within their concep-tualisation of EBP. Sackett, one of the seminal writers in this field, defines EBP as 'the conscientious, explicit and judicious use of current best evidence in making decisions about the care of individual patients . . . integrating with . . . individual expertise and the patient's values and expectations' (Sackett *et al.* 1996).

So, at the point of decision, the practitioner still has to evaluate issues such as:

- the extent to which the current situation matches that envisaged by the studies that generated the evidence
- the extent to which the desired outcomes match those that EBP is aimed at
- the availability of resources and conditions necessary to replicate the circum-stances under which the evidence was generated
- the opportunity cost of carrying out the EBP programme in terms of resources diverted from other procedures or other demands on the service.

So the core of professionalism lies in being able to evaluate evidence in relation to the context rather than just the ability to apply it – what Schön, cited in Chapter 10, calls 'knowing-in-action'.

In Chapter 10, we see that rational models exist along a continuum with other approaches (p. 69ff) and that the context affects the approach of choice. It could be argued, for example, that models of decision making as a conscious and deliberative process are most applicable to the macro levels of prioritisation that set the guidelines and frameworks within which the clinician operates, but on a day-to-day micro level these are likely to be largely internalised and interpreted in relation to the situation at hand and more likely to be at the intuitive end of the continuum. In this context, another concept, again derived from Simon, is useful: that of 'programmability':

> Decisions are programmed to the extent that they are repetitive and routine, to the extent that a definite procedure has been worked out for handling them so that they don't have to be treated from scratch each time they occur.

Decisions on the other hand are non-programmed 'to the extent that they are novel, unstructured and unusually consequential' (Simon 1977, p. 46).

In the healthcare context, we can see that there is a tension between managers and practitioners. Those who manage the service from government down to the level of the individual clinic seek to programme so that strategies relating to fairness and accountability can be adhered to; the individual practitioner is faced with a caseload, much of which exemplifies the unprogrammable. Most of the methods for supporting decision making are understandably aimed at the programmable. It may be that that the non-programmable are inherently unsuited to methodological approaches. That does not mean that decision theory has nothing to offer the individual healthcare professional. Some portions of the role may be 'programmable', at least to some extent, and supporting the decision load for these would be valuable. Even in the least programmable circumstances, having a framework that you are consciously deviating from may at least be helpful in supporting a critically self-reflective approach.

Can prioritisation be fair?

Whether or not prioritisation is methodologically supported, the process results in the allocating of resources to some and the denying of those same resources to others. This raises issues of fairness and justice. Indeed the level of 'fairness' achieved is arguably the only valid way of measuring or evaluating any process of prioritisation; otherwise we could merely operate a 'first come first served' policy in all cases. It could be argued that this is an over-simplification since prioritisation can enable the implementation of complex policies, based on a wide range of considerations, but these policies and strategies are themselves vehicles for the application of what amount to systems of values relating to fairness: even 'first come first served' is a moral position.

Most practitioners are painfully (often literally) aware of the moral complexity of the prioritisation decisions they make – balancing preventative interventions against management of existing disability; the pre-booked client against the unexpected emergency; the potential for natural recovery against the risk of deterioration.

The discipline of moral philosophy has identified and explored a range of possible alternative approaches to the ethics of decision making. By being aware of the extent to which the decision maker is conforming to or deviating from these, the process becomes, if not absolutely accountable, at least coherently debatable. Given that thousands of years of intellectual effort are devoted to the topic, it impossible to do it justice here, but a brief account of some of the major strands may point the way to more comprehensive resources.

Although there are many approaches to ethics, four main strands can be identified: duty-based theories, utilitarian theories, contract-based theories and virtue-based theories. Very briefly, duty-based theories argue that actions are either right or wrong and the criteria for judging this can be codified in some way. This is the basis of most religions and their 'commandments'. Kant (as discussed in Broad 1978) extended this approach by developing the notion of the 'categorical imperative' whereby in a situation not specifically covered by the code, a moral person would act in a way they would wish others to act if they themselves were the recipient of the consequences of the act. This was felt by some to be too inflexible, and Bentham and Stuart Mill amongst others (outlined in Shaw 1999) developed what became known as Utilitarianism in which the focus moved from the act to the consequences of the act and the main guidance was to act in such a way that led to the greatest happiness for the greatest number. Hobbes (from Sorrell 1996) took a rather gloomy view of human nature and argued that people are only obliged to act in a particular way if they have a contractual relation of some kind with the recipient. Otherwise they should do as they wish since fairness consists simply of adhering to agreements.

The virtue approach, which can be traced back to Aristotle, focuses on the person and argues that if people are brought up to be good then they will act in a virtuous way without any need of codes, contracts or moral calculus. Thus it can be seen that the theories variously focus on: the decision itself; the consequences of the decision; the relationship between the decision maker and the other party; and the decision maker himself or herself.

As indicated above, many writers have explored the ethics of rationing in greater detail (e.g. Butler 1999) with particular reference to the issues associated with fair distribution of resources within healthcare. Campbell (2003) contrasts two competing approaches: 'minimum individual entitlement' and 'maximising health gains'. The first suggests that there are some fundamental rights which should be provided for all, equally across all disease groups, and is related to the severity of the condition or on the basis of need. The second focuses not on severity of need but on likelihood of benefit, relative to cost. This approach is consistent with Utilitarianism described above.

These theories are not presented as possible candidates for generating solutions to issues of prioritisation but, given that debates about priorities are often complex and necessarily polemic to some extent, then awareness of such frameworks may well serve to clarify positions and make any assumptions more readily visible and testable.

So what can the practitioner do?

Most of the attention that has been directed at prioritisation in a healthcare context has focused on policy setting at the strategic and management levels. This has come into sharper focus in recent years as information technology has enabled data to be captured and analysed with sufficient speed and economy to make it feasible for policies and targets to be created and monitored virtually in real time. Previously, capturing the necessary data was so expensive that there was a *de facto* recourse to the 'virtue' approach to ethical practice – 'trust me, I'm a doctor'. The increased transparency and accountability of recent years has seen a shift to a more centralised approach to policy making, often centred around achieving measurable performance targets which may be set and evaluated by politicians or managers rather than practitioners.

However even in these circumstances, there is still substantial scope for dis-cretion in prioritisation at the practitioner level, as we have seen from some of the preceding chapters. Looked at from the individual practitioner's perspective, prioritisation is a complex and uncertain process which is largely judgementally based and involves juggling different and sometimes conflicting prioritisation criteria. Each decision relating to an individual client will have implications for other possible ways of treating that client, for other clients on the caseload, for others in the team, as well as for managers responsible for achieving targets at the policy level. Increasingly this is also likely be a collaborative process involving some elements of negotiation with the client or client agents such as parents, as well as with colleagues and immediate supervisors.

In day-to-day practice, it may be that the decision to prioritise or not may not achieve salience in the practitioner's own mind but may be absorbed seamlessly in the flow of events and indeed may even be determined by other decisions made relating to treatment which were not conceived of as being part of a prioritisation process. However such 'decisions' should not be regarded as guesswork or a lack of concern for the issues. It is more a natural result of the increasing use of tacit knowledge and the increasing richness of the clinician's store of such knowledge as expertise develops. The issue then becomes how to ensure that these quasi-intuitive processes continue to work in the best interests of all concerned and as far as possible to monitor the quality of such decisions. The hunch-based process of expertise is actually based on reasoning processes as discussed in Dreyfus and Dreyfus cited in Chapter 10. If we can unpick the key components, then deliberate surfacing of the key elements and ensuring that these are compatible with best practice may be a way of improving prioritisation performance at this micro level. In-service courses, focus groups and possibly increased teamworking may all be ways of achieving this.

Many other authors writing about prioritisation at the macro level recommend a similar exposure of the debate to scrutiny, arguing that, since definitive criteria are not likely to be forthcoming, the movement should be towards progressively more explicit processes. The Rationing Agenda Group (New 1996), while their position supports the use of explicit principles in rationing, draws attention to the fact that not all agree with a principle of explicitness. From this perspective, there is concern that, given the difficulty of achieving methodological and morally sound rationing, public trust in healthcare would be diminished by an open acknowledge-ment of such difficulties, although there is evidence that public confidence in healthcare grows if there is improved information (Coote *et al.* cited in Lenaghan 1997). The parents in our case studies would certainly support that view.

What can prioritisation achieve?

In a world where resources are finite and the potential demand for healthcare potentially infinite, it is not realistic to expect any system of prioritisation to 'solve' the problem of resource allocation. If we are concerned about issues of fairness and effectiveness then some attempt at prioritisation is inescapable and perhaps the greatest contributions that discussion of the issues can make is to identify the range of options and foster critical reflection about our practice. Underpinning any system of prioritisation is a philosophical stance about what is important and what is fair. However, this is often unstated and implicit and even those applying the process may not be consciously aware of this basis.

Arguably, goals should be clear and explicit, especially if we are concerned to allow a range of stakeholders to have a say in the process. Practitioners, clients, and politicians are all key players and transparency is essential for constructive engagement, but attempts at transparency may actually hide more than they reveal. For example, it is attractive to base decisions on measurable outcomes or some kind of points system for severity, such as that described in Withers (1993) in the first chapter. This endeavour is often reflected in the language we use when describing decisions 'weighing up', 'on balance', 'taking into account'; all of which imply a sense of objectivity based on measurement. Dowie (2003) in fact uses the term 'TIABIM – taking into account and bearing in mind' to describe traditional methods of decision making as reflecting this. However when we unpick these processes they become less 'objective'. The numbers frequently represent an essentially subjective weighting and this is particularly significant when we attempt to apply some kind of numeric value to psychosocial factors such as depression or social participation. This is not to argue that numerically based techniques are not useful but that we need to be aware of their dangers, including the spurious air of objectivity that they may bestow, which lay people may be ill-equipped to challenge, and the danger of privileging that which is measurable and neglecting that which is not.

Conclusions

This chapter has identified a number of issues from the preceding chapters – areas of concern in the process of prioritisation. Rather than try to provide solutions to these issues, we have discussed each theme as a set of potential questions for which there are no straightforward answers. Although tempted into drawing final conclusions and making recommendations, we have tried to hold back and present various angles and perspectives on the issues. In the drive to better understand the process of prioritisation we prefer to leave the answers questioned.

References

Broad, C.D. (1978) *Kant: An Introduction*. Cambridge: Cambridge University Press.
Burton, M. and Chapman, M.J. (2004) 'Problems of evidence-based practice in community based services', *Journal of Learning Disabilities*, **8(1)**: 56–70.
Campbell, A. (2003) 'NICE or nasty? Threats to justices from an emphasis on effectiveness', in A. Oliver (ed.) *Health Care Priority Setting: Implications for Health*

Inequalities. Proceedings from a meeting of the Health Equity Network. London: The Nuffield Trust.

Chard, J. (2005) *Taking patients' and clinicians' questions seriously about the effects of treatment*. Paper presented at the James Lind Alliance meeting, 3rd December 2005.

Dowie, J. (2003) 'NICE (and the NHS) – Quo Vadis?' in A. Oliver (ed.) *Health Care Priority Setting: Implications for Health Inequalities*. Proceedings from a meeting of the Health Equity Network. London: The Nuffield Trust.

Irvine, D.H. and Donaldson, L.J. (1995) 'The doctors dilemma', *British Medical Bulletin* **51(4)**: 842–53.

Lenaghan, J. (1997) 'The rationing debate: central government should have a greater role in rationing decisions – the case for', *British Medical Journal*, **314**: 967.

New, B. (1996) 'The rationing agenda in the NHS', *British Medical Journal*, **312**: 1593–601.

Rycroft-Malone, J., Seers, K., Titchen, A., Harvey, G., Kitson, A. and McCormack, B. (2004) 'What counts as evidence in evidence-based practice?' *Journal of Advanced Nursing*, **47(1)**: 81–90.

Sackett, D., Rosenberg, W., Muir-Gray, J., Haynes R., and Richardson, W. (1996) 'Evidence-based medicine – what it is and what it isn't', *British Medical Journal*, **312**: 71–2.

Shaw, William (1999) *Contemporary Ethics: Taking Account of Utilitarianism*. Cambridge, MA: Blackwell.

Shickle, D. (1997) 'Public preferences for health care: prioritisation in the United Kingdom', *Bioethics*, **11(3&4)**.

Simon, H.A. (1977) *The New Science of Management Decision*. New Jersey: Prentice Hall.

Sorrell, T. (ed.) (1996) *The Cambridge Companion to Hobbes*. Cambridge: Cambridge University Press.

Van der Gaag, A., Davis, S., Smith, L. and Mowlese, C. (2003) *Reflections on evidence: an evaluation of therapy and support services for people with aphasia at Connect – the Communication Disability Network, London, UK*. Paper presented at the Comité Permanent de Liaison des Orthophonistes/ Logopèdes de l'Union Européenne Conference, Edinburgh, 2003. www.cplol.org/cplol2003/EN/Full_text_EN/Session1_2_Van_deer_Gaag.htm 30.04.06

Weale, A. (1995) 'The ethics of rationing', *British Medical Bulletin*, **51(4)**: 831–41.

Withers, P. (1993) 'Making children a priority', *College of Speech and Language Therapists Bulletin*, **489**: 12–13.

Chapter 14

Conclusions

Sue Roulstone

The original impetus for this book started many years ago when as a practitioner-manager, I was struggling to make ends meet, to respond to complaints about waiting lists and lack of speech and language therapy services. Editing this book has been part of my quest to develop my understanding of the issues involved in the decisions we make in planning and providing services to children. Throughout my research and underpinning this book, my position has been that practitioners develop understanding and expertise that, if unpicked and discussed, can inform a wider audience.

I am now a researcher, but my approach to knowledge acquisition and research methodology reflects my clinical roots as a speech and language therapist. Like many of my profession, I am an eclectic gatherer of views and perspectives. Speech and language therapists draw on a wide range of disciplines for their epistemologies, for their evidence base: linguists, psychologists, neurologists to name but a few. The profession adopts and adapts the theories of others in order to shed light and find new ways of understanding the disorders and difficulties of people with communication impairments.

The aim of this book has been to explore prioritisation in child health, to open up the debate about what happens in practice in order to better understand what is happening. The goal is always to improve and, although I am wary of becoming what Loughlin in Chapter 9 called the Boss's Helper or the Self-Help Therapist, the book aims to give readers ways of thinking about prioritisation that will stimulate change. In some cases, this might be encouragement to challenge the system, being explicit about the prioritisation that is occurring, collecting data and amassing evidence that can back new funding; in others it might have provided a new insight or way of thinking about decision making that gives confidence and a feeling of being back in control. I hope that it leads to new partnerships where people share the responsibility for making these decisions and to a more open debate with the families and children themselves.

Consideration of the contributions of all the preceding 'data' chapter of Parts II and III generated a number of themes. First, practitioners and parents are trying to make sense of the child health situation. The fight for resources as a parent and the struggle to manage scant resources by practitioners is seen by both as a problem that somehow they must solve. There is a sense that, if only they can find the right solution, somehow the problem will be resolved. However, the overall tenor of the book is that the problem is not likely to go away in the short term. And if we're not careful, reorganising one part of the organisation leads to problems in another.

Issues of power and control were threaded through many of the accounts. Parents feel powerless when they can't get practitioners to listen to them; practitioners feel more confident and in control when they pull back from an abyss of escalating and unmanageable demands; this is in the context of a general lack of clarity about who holds responsibility for making which decisions at which levels. The goals of prioritisation and exactly which agenda or whose agenda they serve is rarely explicit, never mind the criteria upon which subsequent decisions are made. Yet unless we are clear about some of the underlying reasons that drive our activity, there can be little progress towards power sharing and partnership between families and practitioners.

From our practitioners, our parents and our theory writers, we have ideas about tools and strategies that might improve things. As well as resources for their child, parents are looking for openness, honesty and clarity in their dealings with practitioners, for a sense of continuity where they can relax and believe that their children's needs will be met without a continual fight. Our practitioners show us how they have tackled a number of different situations in which resources have been short; they share the criteria and approaches that they have found valuable. Practitioners strive to plan services and strategies for allocating resources in a fair and equitable fashion. Our theory authors provide perspectives from their very different disciplines, different ways of looking at the situation, different tools to use, different concepts which can be used to describe the players in this process, and different criteria for making decisions. From all this we see the complexity and variability of the issues that we all face in meeting the health needs of children.

By this stage in the book, I expect (hope!) that you have ceased to expect a neat set of criteria or principles upon which to base your decisions, although, I agree, that would have been nice! However, even a deceptively simple goal such as making any prioritisation process open and explicit does not have universal support and it is clearly a difficult goal. There are many aspects of the decisions to make explicit and we don't always understand the components ourselves.

I think there are some conclusions that we can extract at a very simple level: an individual practitioner and front-line services will always have to prioritise and manage their day and organise their service, interpreting national level rationing at the level of the individual child and family and locality. We have concluded that single professionals shouldn't take single ownership of the problem to prioritise: even where the decision is about an individual child and family, this needs an honest discussion with the family. Where the decisions are at a service level, then the identification of potential knock-on effects for other services and possible joint solutions should be a consideration. We have explored a range of decision-making approaches and ways of analysing and reflecting upon decisions, and recognised that the context of a decision will impact upon the level of analysis that is possible, while supporting a move towards openness and explicit discussion of prioritisation.

We should not underestimate the complexity of the situation and it seems reasonable to try and equip practitioners with the tools – practical, intellectual and emotional – to deal with prioritisation decisions appropriately. The concepts and fields covered in this book are not a typical part of undergraduate or pre-qualification courses for healthcare practitioners and perhaps it is unreasonable to expect students who are not yet having to make prioritisation decisions with children and families to grapple with the debate. But part of our role as competent practitioners is to understand the limits of our remit and our competence. Understanding the different kinds of prioritisation decisions that are made and at what level in an organisation enables a practitioner to act appropriately and confidently.

Although focusing at a micro level, the issues and concerns are similar to those discussed within the macro-level literature. It is amazingly difficult and contentious to focus at the micro level. To ignore the broader context and to focus on the everyday lives of practitioners suggests a criticism of practitioners when the allocation of resources at a macro level might bring about a solution. But while waiting for the revolution in world economics, practitioners carry on prioritising. This book is not trying to provide a definitive answer and maybe we are doing no more than Loughlin accuses academics of doing: stating the obvious and common sense. But hopefully it has opened the debate on micro-level prioritisation, looking at the impact of rationing at the front line, what it is like for practitioners, examining the realms of what is happening and what is possible.

Index